Patients Beyond Borders Series™

Patients Beyond Borders
Taiwan Edition™

Everybody's Guide to Affordable,
World-Class Medical Travel™

Josef Woodman

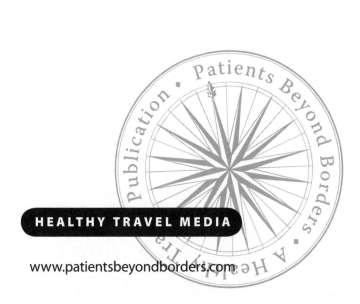

HEALTHY TRAVEL MEDIA

www.patientsbeyondborders.com

PATIENTS BEYOND BORDERS: TAIWAN EDITION
Everybody's Guide to Affordable, World-Class Medical Travel

Copyright © 2008 by Josef Woodman

ISBN 13: 978-0-9791079-3-1

Cover art and page design: Anne Winslow
Developmental Editing: Faith Brynie
Copy Editing: Kate Johnson
Proofreading: Barbara Resch
Indexing: Madge Walls
Typesetting and Production: Copperline Book Services
POD Printing: Catawba Publishing, LLC
Offset Printing: C&C Offset Printing Co, LTD

Printed in China

Healthy Travel Media
P.O. Box 17057
Chapel Hill NC 27516
919 370.7380
info@healthtraveler.net
www.patientsbeyondborders.com

To the Dedicated Healthcare Workers of Taiwan

Limits of Liability and Disclaimer of Warranty
Please Read Carefully

ACKNOWLEDGMENTS

NEARLY FIVE YEARS and the collaboration of hundreds of patients, practitioners, providers, and institutions went into the creation of *Patients Beyond Borders* and its growing library of sister publications, including the *Taiwan Edition* you are holding in your hands.

The history of this series goes back so far that it's hard to know where to begin in expressing thanks. High on the list is literary agent Peter Beren, whose tireless energy and encouragement breathed life into my first efforts in the series. Gerald and Kathleen Hill contributed greatly to the early research. I am grateful to the dozens of gracious professionals at the Apollo Hospitals in India who helped me gain an understanding of the important health considerations behind any medical journey. Special thanks to Anil Maini, Sunita Reddy, and the consummate surgeon Vijay Bose. Also to Doug and Anne Stoda, whose courageous medical trip helped me to locate the true voice and audience for what became the First Edition of *Patients Beyond Borders*.

Today *Patients Beyond Borders* has grown to provide information on hospitals and clinics in 21 countries around the world. For helping me expand the vision as I worked on the Second Edition, I am grateful for the many insights and observations of Jason Yap of Singapore Medicine; Dan Snyder of Parkway in Singapore; Vishal Bali of Wockhardt Hospitals in India; Curtis

Schroeder and Mack Banner of Bumrungrad Hospital in Thailand; James Bae of the Korea Health Industry Development Institute in South Korea; and Steven Tucker of the West Excellence Clinic in Singapore. Deep thanks also to David Boucher, Avery Comarow, Sharon Kleefield, and Karen Timmons for their pearls of wisdom, which led to new paths of research.

This *Taiwan Edition* is the brainchild of the Taiwan Task Force on Medical Travel (TTFMT) and has been realized through the vision of its Secretary General, Dr. Mingyen Wu. Charged with the challenges of helping to unite hospitals and clinics within Taiwan and of bringing new standards of healthcare and international patient services to the country, Dr. Wu faces his daunting task with aplomb. I greatly enjoyed sharing his vision and passion throughout the production of this book. A warm and special thanks to Sherine Kuo and the entire staff at TTFMT. Their tireless efforts and meticulous attention to editorial and medical detail helped bring this informative *Taiwan Edition* to the world.

Finally, a heartfelt note of appreciation to the copyeditors, proofreaders, and indexers who made the *Taiwan Edition* possible. Special thanks to our Editorial Director, Faith Brynie, who hammered the manuscript into a readable, accessible form; and to copyeditor Kate Johnson, who polished these pages and did them proud.

Josef Woodman
Chapel Hill, NC
2008

Contents

PART TWO: TAIWAN'S MOST-TRAVELED HEALTH DESTINATIONS

PART THREE: TRAVELING IN TAIWAN

PART FOUR: RESOURCES AND REFERENCES

PREFACE TO THE TAIWAN EDITION

IN LATE 2007 — less than a year after the publication of the World Edition of *Patients Beyond Borders* — I traveled to Taiwan to gain firsthand experience of medical travel in a country that is arguably one of Asia's best-kept healthcare secrets. I was greeted by a first-world nation, modern bustling cities, relentlessly hard-working people, high-speed bullet trains traversing the country, and — above all — dozens of first-rate medical facilities — universities, research centers, health parks, and more — that would do any medical destination proud.

As you will read in these pages, Taiwan is quickly becoming a bona fide member of the "rising global healthcare tiger" that's beginning to tip the sovereign scales of Western medical practice, offering a world of new choices in affordable care to patients everywhere. Thus, good reasons now abound for millions — if not hundreds of millions — of patients to appreciate Taiwan's medical offerings.

For patients from mainland China, for example, as a rising middle class outstrips that nation's ability to provide quality healthcare, nearby Taiwan offers a convenient and viable alternative. For Hong Kong, Macau, Japan, and neighboring countries that carry high and ever-increasing healthcare costs, Taiwan becomes an attractive destination. In the US, for millions of Chinese Americans without health insurance, a trip to culturally friendly Taiwan can help take some of the financial sting out of an expensive medical procedure. And English-speaking patients will appreciate an increasing effort on the part of the Taiwanese healthcare community to woo a Western clientele into its fold.

Whether patients, physicians, or payers — and regardless of nationality — we are all squarely in the midst of a long overdue revolution: the globalization of healthcare. Although a relative newcomer in this arena, Taiwan is very much a player on the worldwide healthcare front, and the country's influence will become increasingly apparent in all areas of medical care, including research, manufacturing, healthcare services, and more. I hope this *Taiwan Edition* does justice to Taiwan's significant contributions to today's worldwide medical care.

The *Patients Beyond Borders: Taiwan Edition* would not have been possible without the vision and dogged perseverance of Dr. Mingyen Wu of the Taiwan Task Force on Medical Travel. In the early formation of the book, he and I traded dozens of delightful, time-zone-challenged email messages, and his demands for clarity of vision helped to shape the tone and direction of this edition. The Task Force's Research Assistant, Sherine Kuo, courageously absorbed the usual abuse of a book project and managed it with great equanimity and panache. Our Editorial Director, Faith Brynie, provided much-needed guidance, organization, and developmental rigor to the project. Copyeditor Kate Johnson hammered and polished these pages and did them proud. My deepest thanks to them and to all involved in this exciting endeavor.

Josef Woodman

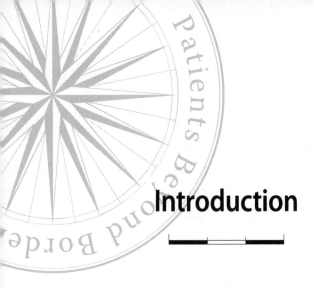

Introduction

Beginnings

The seeds of *Patients Beyond Borders* were sown nearly five years ago, when my father, age 72 at the time, traveled to Mexico for extensive dental work. I well remember my first reaction upon hearing his plans: a mixture of bewilderment and fear, then resignation, knowing that despite my protestations, he was going anyway.

In spite of my concerns — some of them quite real — I'm pleased to report a happy ending. Dad and his wife, Alinda, selected a US-trained dentist in Puerto Vallarta and spent around $11,000 — which included two weeks noodling around the Pacific Coast. They returned tanned and smiling, Dad with new pearly whites and Alinda with an impromptu skin resurfacing. The same procedures would have cost them $24,000 in the US.

After his treatment, when I told the story of my father's trip, most friends responded with the same shock and disbelief that I had felt initially. Then when I explained the quality of care and the savings, more often than not those same folks followed me out the door, asking for Dad's email address. I even had an airport customs agent abandon his post and follow me to the boarding gate, seeking additional information for his son, who he had just learned required heart surgery.

Not long afterward I developed an infected root canal and found myself following my father's example. My research led me abroad for extraction and implant work. While pleasantly surprised at the quality of care, the prices, and the all-around good experience of the trip, I nonetheless made a number of mistakes and created unnecessary difficulties and discomforts for myself. Had I done some simple things differently, my trip would have been more successful and more economical.

In seeking additional data on medical travel, I found no reliable source of information. Everybody had something to sell or a political axe to grind. Books, magazine articles, and newspaper reports seemed more like tourists' brochures than health-travel references. Thus, the idea for *Patients Beyond Borders* was born: a well-researched guide, written in plain English, which would offer an impartial look at contemporary medical travel, while helping prospective patients ask the right questions and make informed choices.

As we contemplate our options in an overburdened global healthcare environment, nearly all of us will eventually find ourselves seeking alternatives to costly treatments — either for ourselves or for our loved ones. Healthcare consumers everywhere are in the midst of a global shift in medical service: in a few short years, big government investment, corporate partnerships, and increased media attention have spawned a new industry—medical tourism—bringing with it a host of encouraging new choices, ranging from dental care and cosmetic surgery to some of the more costly procedures, such as hip replacement and heart surgery. Those patients who take the time to become informed about our changing healthcare world will be pleasantly surprised by the smorgasbord of affordable, high-quality medical options abroad. Those who do not may find themselves grappling with an ungainly, prohibitively expensive healthcare system and a rising absence of choice.

There is no single type of health traveler. In researching and writing *Patients Beyond Borders*, I talked with wealthy women from Beverly Hills who, despite their affluence, prefer the quality of treatment and attention they receive in Brazil or South Africa to medical care California-style. I met a hardworking couple from Wisconsin who, facing the prospect of refinancing their home for a hip operation here in the US, headed to India instead. I interviewed a Vietnam vet who wearied of long waits and red tape. He said "bon voyage" to this country's ever-deteriorating healthcare system and headed overseas for treatment.

After a visit last year to many of Taiwan's fine hospitals and clinics and after lengthy discussions with healthcare administrators and hospital CEOs, it was evident to me that Taiwan ranked high—and deservedly so—as a leading medical travel destination. The all-important combination of attractive pricing with high-quality medical care and related services should soon bring Taiwan to the forefront. Thus, I've prepared this special Taiwan edition of *Patients Beyond Borders* to share what I've learned about Taiwan and relate the experiences of some health travelers who've been treated there.

From these patients' experiences and many more like them, you'll learn when and how health travel to Taiwan might meet your medical and financial needs. And you'll become a more informed healthcare consumer — both here and abroad.

You Deserve an Impartial Perspective

This new phenomenon of medical tourism — or international health travel — has received a good deal of wide-eyed attention of late. While one newspaper or blog giddily touts the fun 'n sun side of treatment abroad, another issues dire warnings about filthy hospitals, shady treatment practices, and procedures gone bad. As with most things in life, the truth lies somewhere in between.

In short, I've found the term "medical tourism" to be something of a misnomer, often leading patients to emphasize the recreational more than the procedural in their quest for medical care abroad. Unlike much of the hype that surrounds contemporary health travel, *Patients Beyond Borders* focuses more on your health than on your travel preferences. Thus, throughout this book, you won't see many references to the terms "medical tourism" or "health tourism." In the same way business travelers don't normally consider themselves tourists, you'll begin to think more in terms of medical travel and health travel.

My research, including countless interviews, has convinced me: with diligence, perseverance, and good information, patients considering traveling abroad for treatment do indeed have legitimate, safe choices, not to mention an opportunity to save thousands of dollars compared to the same treatment at home. Hundreds of patients who have returned from successful treatment overseas provide overwhelmingly positive feedback. They first persuaded me to write the World Edition of *Patients Beyond Borders* as an impartial, scrutinizing guide to becoming an informed international patient. I then designed

> Currently, at least 28 countries on four continents cater to the international health traveler, with more than 2 million patients visiting hospitals and clinics each year in countries other than their own.

this specialized book to help readers reach their own conclusions about whether to seek treatment options in Taiwan.

What Exactly *Is* Medical Tourism?

Last year more than 180,000 Americans, Canadians, and Europeans packed their bags and headed overseas for nearly every imaginable type of medical treatment: knee replacements in India, addiction recovery in Antigua, or restorative dentistry in Mexico. Currently, at least 28 countries on four continents cater to the international health traveler, with more than 2 million patients visiting hospitals and clinics each year in countries other than their own: Indonesians and Cambodians flock to Singapore. Middle Easterners travel to Malaysia and India. Japanese and Chinese journey to Taiwan. In fact, health travelers from all over the world are traveling to Taiwan by the thousands for heart valve replacement, coronary bypass surgery, gastric bypass, joint replacement, hip resurfacing, and more. The roster of treatments is as varied as the travelers.

If the notion of complex medical procedures in far-flung lands seems intimidating to you, don't feel alone. That's why I wrote this book, drawing from the varied experiences of hundreds of patients who, for dozens of reasons, have beaten a well-worn path to successful treatments in Taiwan and other countries.

Why Go Abroad for Medical Care?

Cost savings. Most people like to get the most for their dollar. The single biggest reason patients travel to other countries for medical treatment is the opportunity to save money. Depending upon the country and type of treatment, uninsured and underinsured patients as well as those seeking elective care can realize 15 – 85 percent savings over the cost of treatment at home. Or, as one successful health traveler put it, "I took out my credit card instead of a second mortgage."

> If the notion of complex medical procedures in far-flung lands seems intimidating to you, don't feel alone.

As citizens in the US and other affluent societies reach middle age and beyond, healthcare and prescription costs are devouring nearly 30 percent of retirement and pre-retirement incomes. With the word getting out about top-quality treatments at deep discounts in Taiwan and other nations, informed patients are finding creative alternatives abroad.

Big Surgeries: Comparative Costs Estimates
(All Prices in US Dollars)*

Procedure	US Cost	India	Thailand	Singapore	Malaysia	South Korea	Taiwan
Heart Bypass	$70,000– 133,000	$7,000	$22,000	$16,300	$12,000	$31,750	$25,000– 27,500
Heart Valve Replacement with Bypass	$75,000– 140,000	$9,500	$25,000	$22,000	$13,400	$42,000	$30,000
Hip Replacement	$33,000– 57,000	$10,200	$12,700	$12,000	$7,500	$10,600	$8,800– 9,100
Knee Replacement	$30,000– 53,000	$9,200	$11,500	$9,600	$12,000	$11,800	$9,750– 10,000
Facelift	$10,500– 16,000	$4,800	$5,000	$7,500	$6,400	$6,650	$5,000– 10,000
Gastric Bypass	$35,000– 52,000	$9,300	$13,000	$16,500	$12,700	$9,300	$10,200
Prostate Surgery (TURP)	$10,000– 16,000	$3,600	$4,400	$5,300	$4,600	$3,150	$2,750

*The cost estimates in the table are for surgery, including the hospital stay in a private, single-bed room. Airfare and lodging costs are governed by individual preferences. To compute a ballpark estimate of total costs, add $5,000 for you and a companion, as an approximation of coach airfare and hotel rooms averaging $150 per night. So the cost of coronary bypass surgery in Taiwan might total about $32,500 — an estimated savings of from $37,500 to $100,500 compared to the cost in the US. Individual situations vary widely, however, so be sure to get firm numbers from healthcare providers, both at home and abroad, before making any decisions.

Better quality care. Veteran health travelers know that facilities, instrumentation, and customer service in treatment centers abroad often equal or exceed those found in the US. In fact, governments of countries such as Taiwan have poured billions of dollars into improving their healthcare systems, which are now aggressively catering to the international health traveler. VIP waiting lounges, deluxe hospital suites, and staffed recuperation resorts are common amenities, along with free transportation to and from airports, low-cost meal plans for companions, and discounted rates at hotels affiliated with the hospital.

Moreover, physicians and staff in treatment centers abroad are often far more accessible than medical personnel back home. It's not unusual for physicians and surgeons to give patients their cell phone numbers to ensure immediate contact, especially during the post-treatment recovery period.

Excluded treatments. Even the most robust health insurance plans exclude a variety of conditions and treatments. You, the policyholder, must pay these expenses out-of-pocket. Although health insurance policies vary according to the underwriter and individual, your plan probably excludes a variety of treatments, such as cosmetic surgeries, dental care, vision treatments, reproductive/infertility procedures, certain non-emergency cardiovascular and orthopedic surgeries, weight-loss programs, substance-abuse rehabilitation, and prosthetics — to name only a few. In addition, many policies place restrictions on prescriptions (some quite expensive), post-operative care, congenital disorders, and pre-existing conditions.

Rich or cash-challenged, young or not-so-young, heavily or only lightly insured — folks who get sick or desire a treatment (even one recommended by their physician) often find their insurance won't cover it, leaving millions of patients with financial challenges and a dearth of options in their own country.

Even the most robust health insurance plans exclude a variety of conditions and treatments. You, the policyholder, must pay these expenses out-of-pocket.

Specialty treatments. Some procedures and prescriptions are simply not allowed in a patient's home country. A certain procedure may be disallowed, or perhaps it's still in the testing and clinical trials stage or was only recently approved. Such treatments are often offered abroad.

One example is an orthopedic procedure known as hip resurfacing, which for most patients is a far superior, longer lasting, and less expensive alternative to the traditional hip replacement still practiced almost exclusively in some countries. While this procedure has been performed for more than a decade throughout Europe and Asia, it was only recently approved in the US, where its availability remains spotty and its effective performance unproven. Hundreds of forward-thinking Americans, many having suffered years of chronic pain, have found relief in Asian countries where hip resurfacing techniques, materials, and instrumentation have been perfected and the procedure is routine.

Shorter waiting periods. For decades, thousands of Canadian and British subscribers to universal, "free" healthcare plans have endured waits as long as two years for established procedures. "Some of us die before we get to the operating table,"

> Staff-to-patient ratios are usually lower abroad, as are hospital-borne infection rates.

commented one exasperated patient, who journeyed abroad for an open-heart procedure.

In the US, long waits are a growing problem, particularly among war veterans covered under the Veterans Administration Act, for whom long queues are becoming far too common. Some patients figure it's better to pay out-of-pocket to get out of pain or halt a deteriorating condition than to suffer the anxiety and frustration of waiting for a far-future appointment and other medical uncertainties.

More "inpatient-friendly." As health insurance companies apply increasing pressure on hospitals to move inpatients out of those costly beds as quickly as possible, outpatient procedures are becoming the norm. Medical travelers will welcome the flexibility at the best hospitals abroad, where they are often aggressively encouraged to spend extra time in the hospital post-procedure. Staff-to-patient ratios are usually lower abroad, as are hospital-borne infection rates.

The lure of the new and different. Although traveling abroad for medical care can be challenging, many patients welcome the chance to blaze a trail, and they find the creature comforts often offered abroad to be a welcome relief from the sterile, impersonal hospital environments so frequently encountered at home. For others, simply being in a new and interesting culture lends distraction to an otherwise worrisome, tedious process. And getting away from the myriad obligations of home and professional life can yield healthful effects at a stressful time.

What's more, travel — and particularly international travel — can be a life-changing experience. You might be humbled by the limousine ride from Taiwan Taoyuan International Airport to a hotel in central Taipei, struck by the simple, elegant graciousness of professionals and ordinary people in a foreign land, or wowed by the sheer beauty of the landscape outside the window of a hotel or hospital. Medical travelers can bring back more from their trip than improved health. They can return with an appreciation for a landscape, a culture, and way of life far different from their own.

Who Should Read *Patients Beyond Borders: Taiwan Edition*?

You'll benefit from reading this book if

✦ You're one of the millions of uninsured or underinsured individuals who wish to explore less expensive options for a treatment often covered by health insurance.

✦ You wish to pursue an elective treatment (such as cosmetic surgery, in vitro fertilization, or homeopathy) not normally covered by health insurance.

✦ You're exploring a treatment not offered or not approved in your home country.

✦ You're seeking the benefits of a rich history of traditional Chinese medicine with a backdrop of modern, Westernized medical practice.

✦ You feel a friend or family member might benefit from learning more about health travel, yet that person might lack the confidence or focus to launch an inquiry.

✦ You plan to join a family member or friend for treatment abroad (see Chapter Six, "For Companions").

What *Patients Beyond Borders: Taiwan Edition* Will (and Won't) Do for You

Your condition, diagnosis, treatment options, and travel preferences are unique, and only you — in consultation with your physician and loved ones — can determine the best course of action.

Patients Beyond Borders: Taiwan Edition isn't a guide to medical diagnosis and treatment, nor does it provide medical advice on specific treatments or caregiver referrals. Your condition, diagnosis, treatment options, and travel preferences are unique, and only you — in consultation with your physician and loved ones — can determine the best course of action.

Should you decide to travel to Taiwan for treatment, we *do* provide you with all the resources and tools necessary to become an informed medical traveler, so you'll have the best possible travel experience and treatment your money can buy.

Our job is to

✦ help you become a knowledgeable, confident health traveler;

✦ assist you in planning and budgeting your trip and treatment;

✦ provide you with up-to-date information about the most popular, well-established treatment centers;

✦ help make your visit to Taiwan as comfortable and hassle-free as possible;

✦ recommend good lodging and recovery accommodations; and

✦ provide tips and advice for a successful medical travel experience — before, during, and after treatment.

Your job is to

✦ consult with your local doctor(s) to ensure you've reached a satisfactory diagnosis and recommended course of treatment;

✦ decide, based on your research and the material covered in this book, whether you wish to travel to Taiwan for treatment; and if so,

✦ select a treatment center and physician based on the information you find in this book and elsewhere.

It's a truism: every journey begins with the first step. Health travel is no exception. And once you've taken that first step toward learning more, your friends, family, this book, and a trusty Internet connection will speed you on your way.

How to Use This Book

Before you dive into Part Two, "Taiwan's Most-Traveled Health Destinations," you should carefully read **Part One, "How to Become a Savvy, Informed Medical Traveler."** It provides you with the basic resources and tools you'll need to do your research and make an informed decision.

Chapter One, "What Am I Getting Into? Some Quick Answers for Health Travelers," addresses the questions and concerns most often voiced by patients (and their loved ones) considering a medical journey abroad.

Chapter Two, "Planning Your Health Travel Journey," helps you design your trip step by step. The chapter provides data and advice culled from interviews with hundreds of patients and treatment center personnel. You'll learn how to cut through the chaff quickly to find the right clinics, determine physician qualifications, narrow your destination choices, choose the right companion, and more.

Chapter Three, "Budgeting Your Treatment and Trip," walks you through the financial basics of a medical trip and gives you the tools you need to prepare an estimated budget. Our *"Patients Beyond Borders* Budget Planner" helps you determine specific cost-savings and avoid financial surprises.

Chapter Four, "While You're There," provides valuable information on what to expect from your treatment center and physician, plus general tips for dealing with local culture, language barriers, and more. A section on communicating while on the road provides pointers on using cell phones and computers to communicate with physicians in-country and loved ones back home.

Chapter Five, "Home Again, Home Again," helps you get settled in after your journey is over, offering practical advice on working with your hometown doctor, shaking off the "post-treatment blues," coping with discomforts and complications, and getting back on your feet.

Chapter Six, "For Companions," is written especially for those caring family members or friends who accompany patients on health journeys.

Chapter Seven, "Dos and Don'ts for the Smart Health Traveler," helps you avoid common speed bumps and potholes on the health travel road.

Part Two, "Taiwan's Most-Traveled Health Destinations," features 19 hospitals and clinics in Taiwan, with up-to-date information on treatment specialties, accreditation, transportation, communication, and more. You can use the information in this section to get a good idea about where to travel for your particular procedure and what to expect when you get there.

Part Three, "Traveling in Taiwan," provides basic information that will help you plan your trip to Taiwan. It also describes a few of the sights that attract tourists to this island nation.

Part Four, "Resources and References," provides additional information on medical travel to Taiwan and helpful links, plus a glossary of commonly used medical terms.

As you work your way through decision-making and subsequent planning, remember that you're following in the footsteps of tens of thousands of health travelers who have made the journey before you. The overwhelming majority have returned home successfully treated, with money to spare in their savings accounts.

Still, the process—particularly in the early planning—can be daunting, frustrating, even a little scary. That's normal, and every health traveler we interviewed experienced "the Big Fear" at one time or another. Healthcare abroad is not for everyone, and part of being a smart consumer is evaluating all the impartial data available before making an informed decision. If you accomplish that in reading *Patients Beyond Borders: Taiwan Edition*, we've achieved our mission.

Let's get started.

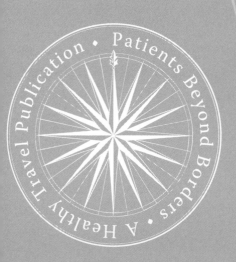

PART ONE

How to Become a Savvy, Informed, Medical Traveler

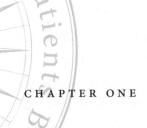

What Am I Getting Into? Some Quick Answers for Health Travelers

Is Healthcare Overseas Safe?

Interestingly, the friends and family members of patients considering healthcare abroad ask this question more often than do the patients themselves. In fact, at least one friend or family member is virtually guaranteed to balk at the thought of your heading overseas for treatment. Most of these concerns are unfounded. They usually arise either from a lack of knowledge or from cultural myopia.

Although no medical procedure is 100 percent risk free anywhere in the world, the best international hospitals and clinics offer quality of care, numbers of surgeries, and success rates equal to the best hospitals in the US, UK, and Europe. In fact, many hospitals abroad are accredited by the same agency (the Joint Commission) that certifies hospitals in the US. (For more information on hospital accreditation and safety standards, see Chapter Two, "Planning Your Health Travel Journey.")

It's not hard to find overseas physicians, dentists, and surgeons who received their medical training and degrees at first-rate medical schools in the US, Great Britain, Canada, Switzerland, or Germany.

Finally, compared to the US, many international hospitals — particularly the larger institutions in Asia — boast lower morbidity rates, especially when it comes to complex cardiac and orthopedic surgeries, for which success rates higher than 98.5 percent are the norm in those countries.

If Healthcare in Other Countries Is So Good, How Can It Be So Cheap?

High running costs of facilities, unpaid hospital bills totaling billions of dollars, high-priced medical education, costly research, and excessive malpractice litigation all add up to exorbitant prices for healthcare in the US and several other nations.

Many hospitals abroad are accredited by the same agency (the Joint Commission) that certifies hospitals in the US.

In addition, physicians who perform elective and specialty procedures — such as cosmetic surgeries, in vitro fertilization, and certain hip, spine and cardiac procedures — often command astronomical fees from patients willing and able to pay, leaving those of more modest means in the lurch and seeking alternatives.

Healthcare in many other countries, however, is less costly because standards of living are more modest, doctors and staff command lower wages, government-subsidized healthcare keeps private healthcare costs down, and malpractice attorneys are, if not docile, at least considerably more restrained.

How Much Can I Save?

Your savings will depend on your treatment, your selected destination, and your travel and lifestyle preferences. Patients who travel to Taiwan might save more than $50,000 on the US price.

A good rule of thumb for medical travel is "the $6,000 Rule": If your specialist quotes you a price of US$6,000

> If your specialist quotes you a price of US$6,000 or more for a treatment, chances are good that one or more foreign countries can offer you the same procedure and quality for less, even including your travel and lodging expenses.

or more for a treatment, chances are good that one or more foreign countries can offer you the same procedure and quality for less, even including your travel and lodging expenses. If your specialist's quote is less than US$6,000, you're probably better off having your treatment at home.

Is It Safe to Travel Overseas?

Your own behavior will determine much of your experience abroad. If you follow the common sense rules of courtesy and observe cultural norms, you should be safe in any country. Outcomes have proven that's true. Hundreds of thousands of international health travelers return home safe and sound each year.

Health travelers can be further reassured because, from the moment of arrival in another country until embarking on a homebound plane, most are under the constant care of a hospital, health travel broker, tour agency, or other third-party agent. Most health travelers are met at their airport arrival gate and whisked to a modern hospital or hotel. From that point, they're usually either under someone's care in a treatment center, getting a bite in a restaurant, or resting in a cozy hotel room.

What Medical Treatments Are Available Abroad?

Although nearly every kind of treatment is possible abroad, most international patients head overseas for orthopedics (hip replacement, knee replacement, spinal work); cardiovascular surgery (bypass, valve replacement, heart transplant); cancer diagnosis and treatment; dental care (usually more extensive cosmetic or restorative work); or cosmetic surgery. In addition, medical travelers seek specialty treatments (such as fertility diagnosis and in vitro fertilization procedures), weight-loss procedures (such as bariatric surgeries), and procedures not yet allowed at home (such as certain stem cell therapies). In Part Two of this book, you'll discover a range of treatment options in Taiwan to match nearly any medical need.

What all those treatments have in common is great expense. The huge savings to be garnered abroad can outweigh the challenges of traveling overseas for treatment.

Can Someone Come Along with Me?
I Don't Like Traveling Alone

That's good, because we don't recommend you travel alone. We've found that most health travelers fare better with a companion in tow — a spouse, family member, or friend. Companions don't greatly increase the overall costs of a trip, and they can actually save you time and money in the end, because they are looking out for your interests every step of the way. For more information on traveling with family or friends, see Chapter Six, "For Companions."

Even if you cannot travel with a companion, or prefer not to, you won't be going it alone in Taiwan. If staying in a hospital, the quality of care and attention you'll receive in the better centers is truly remarkable, with low nurse-to-patient ratios and a host of staffers, orderlies, physician's assistants, and dieticians streaming in and out of your room with great frequency. You'll make fast friends during your stay.

How Realistic Is the "Vacation"
Part of the Trip?

That depends on the type of treatment you're seeking, how much time you have, and how comfortable you feel combining leisure travel with the medical side of your trip. Most patients who take a vacation as part of a health travel journey are either planning to travel anyway or have allocated a good deal of additional time for recreation as well as recovery — there's a big difference, which we cover in Chapter Four, "While You're There."

Throughout this book, we encourage patients to focus more on their treatment and recovery than on tourism, even for the less invasive procedures. Web sites and health travel brochures peppered with zealous promotion ("Enjoy Fabulous Vacation in Taiwan While Recovering from Your Tummy Tuck!") ignore the realities of health travel. Long flights, post-treatment recovery, and just plain being alone in a faraway place can be overwhelming, even for the most optimistic health traveler.

Think of your medical journey more as a business trip than a leisure junket. Consider socking away some of your savings for a separate vacation you and a loved one can take after the primary challenge of managing your immediate health need is behind you. Then, by all means, break out the champagne at a far-flung exotic hideaway and celebrate your health and good fortune.

> We encourage patients to focus more on their treatment and recovery than on tourism.

What If Complications Arise after I Return Home?

Depending on your treatment, your physician or surgeon will usually strongly advise you to stay in Taiwan for at least a few days post-treatment. Your doctor will want to make sure your treatment went well, your medications are working as they should, you're settling into any recommended physical therapies, and your required followups are going according to plan. Thus, by the time you board the plane home, your risk of complications will be greatly reduced.

In the unlikely event that you develop complications after

returning home, you'll need to decide whether to make a repeat trip or continue your treatment at home. Some procedures, such as dental work, are guaranteed; so it may well be financially worthwhile, albeit inconvenient, to return to Taiwan. If you choose not to, most overseas dentists and surgeons are happy to talk with your hometown physician to discuss complications and recommend further action. For more information on complications and other post-treatment considerations, see Chapter Five, "Home Again, Home Again."

Prior to traveling abroad for treatment, be sure to let your local doctor(s) know your plans. It's better to alert them beforehand than to surprise them after the fact. (See "Continuity of Care" in Chapter Two.)

Will My Health Insurance Cover My Medical Expenses in Taiwan?

As of this writing, it's possible, but not probable. While the largest employers and healthcare insurers — not to mention politicians — struggle with new models of coverage, most plans do not yet cover the costs of obtaining treatment abroad. Yet, with healthcare costs threatening to literally bust the economy in some countries, pressures for change are mounting. Recognizing that globalization of healthcare is now a reality, insurers, employers, and hospitals are now beginning to form partnerships with payers and providers in Taiwan and other countries. By the time you read this book, large insurers may already be offering coverage (albeit limited) in Taiwan. Check with your insurer for the latest on your coverage abroad.

Can I Sue?

For better or worse, most countries do not share the Western attitude toward personal and institutional liability. A full discussion of the reasons lies outside the scope of this book. Here's a good rule of thumb: if legal recourse is a primary concern in making your health travel decision, you probably shouldn't head abroad for medical treatment.

If, however, you experience severe complications and fail to receive the followup care you think you need or deserve, then you may want to consider legal action, say attorneys Amanda Hayes and Natasha Bellroth of Global MD. "Legal recourse and remedies are generally limited abroad for patients who experience bad outcomes in foreign facilities," they say. "Moreover, a patient's ability to sue a foreign physician or facility for medical malpractice is limited by the availability of an appropriate forum in which to bring a lawsuit."

For example, say Hayes and Bellroth, assume that American patient John Smith travels to Taiwan for hip replacement surgery and suffers a bad outcome at ABC Hospital that was caused by his surgeon's negligence. Mr. Smith has some options for pursuing a judicial remedy:

- In order to sue ABC Hospital in the United States, a US court must be able to exercise jurisdiction over ABC Hospital, a Taiwanese Corporation with no offices or employees in the United States. US courts may only assert general or specific personal jurisdiction over a foreign entity when the foreign entity's presence or dealings where the suit is brought justify requiring the company to defend suit there.

- Assuming that the case proceeds to judgment against ABC Hospital in the US, Mr. Smith will face an uphill battle to enforce an American judgment in Taiwan. If Mr. Smith won a large punitive damage award from an American court, he would be disappointed to learn that punitive damage awards are rarely awarded outside of the US (another reason for the high cost of healthcare in the US) and are unlikely to be enforced (in any of the countries currently attracting American medial tourists).

- Alternatively, Mr. Smith may try to sue ABC Hospital in Taiwan, which will require that Mr. Smith hire a lawyer in Taiwan and perhaps travel back to Taiwan to attend the proceedings. Even if Mr. Smith prevailed against ABC Hospital in Taiwan, he will probably only be able to recover his actual damages (the provable out-of-pocket cost of harm caused by negligence, e.g., medical bills incurred for corrective surgery and time away from work) since few countries award punitive damages to successful plaintiffs.

- Mr. Smith may seek to arbitrate his claim against ABC Hospital before an international tribunal. For example, the International Court of Arbitration of the International Chamber of Commerce may provide Mr. Smith with a viable and likely more cost efficient way to hold ABC Hospital accountable for its negligence. Generally, an agreement to arbitrate claims must be in place before the relationship commences. Mr. Smith should have confirmed that ABC Hospital had agreed to arbitrate potential future claims and where those proceedings would occur prior to surgery.

Each alternative forum presents its own unique set of challenges. There is no ideal solution that would put judicial recourse against a foreign entity on par with the remedies available against a US hospital or physician. There are, however, practical measures that Mr. Smith might have taken before he traveled to Taiwan that would have helped him to manage the risk in the unlikely event of a bad outcome.

- For example, Mr. Smith might have purchased insurance (your health travel agency should be able to point you to available policies) designed specifically to protect him from the financial consequences of foreseeable complications and unforeseeable medical malpractice. Such insurance could have helped Mr. Smith eliminate the cost of legal action while compensating him up to the amount of the policy limit he purchased.
- In addition, had Mr. Smith paid for his procedure with a major credit card, his card company may have allowed him to recover the cost of a disappointing treatment by disputing the charges.
- Finally, Mr. Smith could have made sure that the health travel agency that planned his procedure had a clear and reasonable protocol in place with the treating facility on how to deal with bad outcomes and complications. Ideally, the hospital will have agreed to absorb costs associated with making Mr. Smith whole again (return flight, accommodations and corrective procedure) and compensate him if he cannot be satisfied.

Ultimately, there is no perfect way to compensate a patient (either domestically or abroad) who has suffered an imperfect outcome after a medical procedure. The good news is that informed patients can take preventive measures to protect themselves before they travel abroad for care so that they are not left in the hands of imperfect healthcare insurance and judicial systems.

Foreign hospitals are eager to prove that they have surgeons and technical facilities with quality that rivals and even exceeds that found in Western nations. Your independent research will reveal that sophisticated foreign hospitals and governments are heavily invested in serving international patients with high-quality healthcare; they understand that the publicity associated with even one bad outcome could quickly end the growing flow of health travelers.

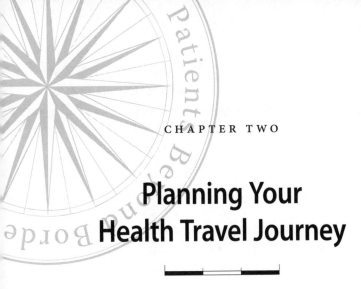

CHAPTER TWO

Planning Your
Health Travel Journey

First Things First: Seek Guidance

As you've probably learned from previous trips, an expert guide can teach you things and take you places you would not have otherwise discovered. Consider Part One of *Patients Beyond Borders: Taiwan Edition* your "health travel planning companion," a trusty sidekick to help ease the burdens of your journey. You'll progress more safely and easily if you draw upon the collective wisdom of those who have traveled successfully before you.

Although each journey varies according to the traveler's preferences and pocketbook, good planning is essential to the success of any trip. That goes double for the medical traveler. In this chapter you'll learn how to become an informed global patient. If you decide that a medical trip is right for you, we'll help you gain confidence about selecting the best clinic and physician and working with others to help ensure your success.

Action Item: **Research several physicians, clinics, or hospitals that offer the treatment you need. Don't snap up the first option you find.**

Trust Yourself

Most likely, you're considering health travel because you want an elective treatment, such as cosmetic surgery or infertility treatment, or because you've been diagnosed with a health problem that requires surgical intervention, such as orthopedic or cardiovascular surgery. Whatever the reason, a condition you want or need treated — usually coupled with a desire or need for substantial cost savings (and for some, a sense of adventure or a wish to try something new) — is what brought you to this point.

Other factors may be influencing your decision as well. It's no secret that contemporary economic and medical trends in many countries have spawned overworked practitioners, crowded hospitals, and vast variations in the quality of care available to all but the wealthiest citizens. Your dad's or grandmother's friendly, chatty, all-knowing family doctor has become a medical oddity, supplanted by a bevy of busy assistants, hurried consultations, arms-length testing, hasty diagnoses, and increasingly inadequate treatment. As a result, the traditional trusting patients of yesteryear, who unquestioningly put their lives in the hands of the medical system, are a rapidly disappearing breed.

Today patients are urged to educate themselves, take a proactive stance, and ask questions. Increasingly, medical systems are based on market principles. This makes you a consumer of healthcare. As a consumer, you should remember "buyer beware" in all your choices.

If you're holding this book in your hand right now, chances are you've left the old world of blind faith and have appropriately adapted to modern medical times, evolving into a curious, assertive, informed patient. Congratulations! Your prognosis for becoming a successful health traveler is vastly improved.

> Plan ahead, as far in advance as you can. Three months prior to treatment is good. Six months ahead of time is great. One month is not so good.

Knowledge is power, and the more thought you put into weighing your options, the more confidence you'll gain in reaching the decision that's best for you and your loved ones. Even if you only skim the rest of this book, read this chapter carefully and thoroughly. At the end of it, you'll have answered enough questions to know whether, when, and where to travel for your medical care.

Plan Ahead

Okay. You're beginning to recover from the heart-stopping quote your medical specialist laid on you two weeks ago. You've talked with friends and family about heading abroad for treatment. They're skeptical but reluctantly willing to trust your judgment. Truth be told, you're still a tad skeptical yourself, but you're willing to consider medical travel as an option.

Long before you pack your bags, you have a lot to do and a logical progression of decisions and events to work through. The first item of business is to plan ahead, as far in advance as you can. Three months prior to treatment is good. Six months ahead of time is great. One month is not so good. Here's why:

✦ **The best overseas physicians are also the busiest.** That's a fact everywhere. Just as here in the US, doctors, surgeons, and specialists abroad work 24/7, and their schedules are often established a month or more in advance. If you want the most qualified doctor and the best care your global patient money can buy, give the doctors and treatment centers you select plenty of time to work you into their calendars.

✦ **The lowest international airfares go to those who book early.** As veteran international travelers know, ticket prices rise savagely as the departure date draws closer. Most punishing of all are last-minute fares, best reserved for family tragedies, rich jetsetters, and busy corporate executives. Booking at least 60 days prior to treatment allows you to avoid the unhappy upward spiral of air travel costs.

If you're planning to redeem frequent-flyer miles, try to book at least 90 days in advance, even if you're not 100 percent certain of your treatment date. At this writing, most airlines don't charge for schedule changes on frequent-flyer fares, and you're better off reserving a date — then changing it later — than being stuck without any reservation at all.

Similarly, for paid fares, it's usually better to reserve your trip as far in advance as you can, giving your best guess at a schedule. Then, budget for the financial penalty in case you need to change your flight itinerary.

✦ *Peak seasons can snarl the best-laid plans.* International tourism is again on the rise. If you want or need to travel during Taiwan's busy tourist season, start planning your health trip four to six months in advance.

✦ *Preparation is a big part of success.* When you paint your living room wall, you know that preparation is half the effort; by the time you pick up the paintbrush, you're halfway done. The same is true with health travel. Before you can book your flight or reserve your hotel room, you must first confirm your treatment appointment. Before you do that, you'll need to decide which hospital you want to go to, which physician(s) suit your needs, and much more.

While such planning is not rocket science, an organized approach in the preparation stages will save you time and money in the end. In the following pages, we provide a guide to that organized approach.

Set Your Mind to It

As you plan, your mindset is as important as any set of skills. So cultivate and practice the following:

An open mind. Our twenty-first-century world is increasingly becoming a global village. Still, contrasts abound: different time zones (they're sleeping while we're working); different accents (English can take on many forms, some of them barely comprehensible to Americans); different clothes; different table manners; and much more. Those with a strictly Western-centric cultural bias may have trouble absorbing and accommodating such diversity. You need an open mind to accept that other points of view and ways of life are not only valid but in some respects perhaps, more refined than yours. After all, Western cultures are adolescent compared to thousands of years of Asian civilization.

Patience. As you embark on your health journey, you'll find that patience is indeed a virtue, particularly in the planning stages.

For one thing, the pace abroad is generally slower — and more cordial. While in the US you might expect your inquiry returned within three hours, you may not hear back from a hospital overseas for three days. Be patient. Call or email a second time. If you don't get an answer in a week, move on. There are plenty of hospitals and clinics in Taiwan willing and able to work with you. Finding the right one is a systematic process, sometimes involving false starts.

> After all, Western cultures are adolescent compared to thousands of years of Asian civilization.

Persistence. When planning any international trip, you'll encounter a host of tasks, contingencies, and sometimes setbacks. So, be flexible but persistent in your planning. If Plan A isn't working, move to Plan B. You'll sometimes find yourself at Plan D, only to discover that Plan B worked out after all, although not on your expected timetable. Generally, the early planning stages require the most perseverance.

Email and Internet Searching

Although you needn't be a computer whiz, you'll gain a huge advantage from an Internet connection for two important purposes:

Communication. As annoying and inefficient as telephones are in daily life, they are exponentially more so when you're trying to conduct business from afar. Email, on the other hand, knows no time zones, lowers the language barrier, and provides an efficient information trail for contacts, recommendations, and myriad other details you'd otherwise be obliged to somehow remember.

Email is vital for making initial inquiries, following up on research, confirming and reconfirming appointments, booking airline and hotel reservations, and keeping records of your transactions with physicians and staff. You needn't be a great journalist or business correspondent; if you can email successfully with your kids or chat it up on Instant Messenger with your sister, you'll do fine.

Research. What a world we live in, where all earthly knowledge is now truly at our fingertips! The rise of the Web and the refinement of search engines, such as Google, MSN, and Yahoo, have enabled anyone with an Internet connection to obtain reliable research results quickly and easily.

Primary to successful health travel planning is a basic ability to gather and sort information. The Internet offers some big keys to the research kingdom. Indeed, ten years ago, medical travel as we know it would have been possible only for those with professional leverage or inside information. Today the power of that knowledge is available to us all.

For some of us, however, these new Internet tools are as bewildering as they are powerful. If you don't like doing the required digging, or if you aren't confident in your research skills, perhaps a family member or friend is willing to help. Make your fact-finding a shared project — perhaps working with a younger member of your circle who can show off his or her computer prowess. Although *Patients Beyond Borders: Taiwan Edition* provides sufficient guidelines to help get anyone started in finding the right fit for particular treatment needs, the specifics of where to go and which doctor to engage are up to the individual. Making such decisions requires doing your homework, and the Internet is a great homework tool.

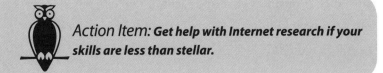

Action Item: **Get help with Internet research if your skills are less than stellar.**

Chutzpah!

During the planning stages, make sure you maintain the will to keep moving forward, the courage to do things a little differently, and the confidence that you're making the right choices. Along your health journey you're likely to encounter local physicians who aren't happy that you're heading overseas for treatment, friends and relatives who think you're nuts (even if they didn't previously), and days of genuine self-doubt. But stick with it. Don't let other people talk you out of your quest because of their ignorance, anxiety, or competitive zeal. If you do your homework and follow the guidelines in this book, you'll make the right decisions.

Look for a Medical Travel Agent

Once upon a time, travel agents arranged trips for everyone, but times have changed, and many of us have now become accustomed to booking our own travel arrangements over the Internet. However, there exists out there a new category of travel agents who have a special set of skills and serve a special purpose: they arrange medical travel. These agents know doctors and hospitals abroad. They can anticipate their clients' needs for transportation and other services when seeking healthcare on foreign soil. Such agents frequently provide "package deals" of treatments, travel, and services that they arrange in advance, often negotiating excellent amenities and bargain-basement prices for their clients — not only with doctors and hospitals, but also with airlines and hotels.

If you don't want to do all your planning on your own, look for a health travel agent who serves Taiwan. An Internet search for <medical tourism>, <health travel agent>, or <medical travel> may turn up several in your home country. Choose your medical travel agent the way you'd choose any other provider: look for experience, competence, and a can-do attitude.

As of this writing, no specialized medical travel agents are established in Taiwan itself. However, some of Taiwan's travel agencies are working to cultivate their expertise in medical tourism, so you may well find new ones popping up just when you need them. Typically, travel agencies in Taiwan offer the usual travel services and then refer medical inquiries to hospital personnel. Although medical and traveling services are usually kept separate in Taiwan, some hospitals do provide travel assistance to international patients, including help with visa applications and local transportation.

Eleven Steps to Enlightened Health Travel Planning

The following is culled from hundreds of interviews with patients and treatment center staff members around the world. Follow the steps and advice outlined here and you'll streamline your planning, organize your trip well, select the best physician(s), communicate effectively with staff, save money, and pack your bags with confidence.

Step 1: Confirm Your Treatment Options

1 Doctors generally recommend a range of choices for a given condition, then leave it up to you and your family to settle upon a course of action based on their recommendations. After all, the buck stops with your body, especially these days, and no one other than you can or should make those important health-related judgment calls. Most physicians respect that, and that's why they usually stop short of advising you what specific course of treatment to take. That's wise, because your body is your own and so are such vital decisions. Most physicians respect their patient's autonomy.

If you have doubts about your diagnosis or feel dissatisfied in your relationship with your physician or specialist, don't be timid about seeking a second — or even third — opinion. At the very least, a second opinion expands your knowledge base about your condition. The more you and your hometown health team learn about — and discuss — your condition, diagnosis, and treatment options, the more precisely and confidently you'll communicate with your overseas practitioners.

Action Item: **Request copies of all local consultations and recommendations in writing, along with cost estimates for treatment. Then begin a file for all paperwork related to your treatment and travel.**

As you sort through your treatment options and consider courses of action, you'll want to learn as much as you can about your condition. You'll get better care from your overseas practitioners if you are a knowledgeable and responsive patient.

It works both ways: your experiences and challenges as an informed medical traveler will also sharpen your skills on the home front, better equipping you and your loved ones to survive and flourish in the increasingly complex morass of our contemporary healthcare system.

Becoming Informed Here and Abroad

Toward becoming the best possible patient both at home and abroad, we highly recommend you buy, beg, or borrow and read — cover to cover — *You: The Smart Patient: An Insider's Guide for Getting the Best Treatment* by Michael F. Roizen and Mehmet C. Oz. These two physicians have written a witty, often irreverent, and highly useful guide to becoming an informed patient, whether in your doctor's office or dentist's chair, on the surgeon's table, or in an emergency room. This 400-page consumer bible is packed with information on patients' rights, surgical precautions, second and third opinions, health insurance plans, health records, and precautionary advice that falls outside the scope of *Patients Beyond Borders: Taiwan Edition*.

Step 2: Narrow Your Destinations

2 Once you've decided what treatment you're seeking and that Taiwan may be the right destination for you, turn to Part Two to review the various hospitals, specialties, and treatments available. Part Two will help you locate the care you are looking for. In addition, you may want to obtain advice from your local doctor, friends, or trusted sources on the Internet.

Your searches are likely to produce a list of several places that offer, for example, excellent cardiac care. Great! Choice is good. You can then narrow your search based on your travel preferences, geography, budget, time requirements, and other variables. To help pare down your options, ask yourself these questions:

✦ When do I want — or need — to travel?

✦ If I'm taking a companion, when can he or she travel?

✦ How much do I mind a ten-hour flight? An 18-hour flight?

✦ Do I have a preference for a season or type of weather?

✦ If I'm planning to enjoy some leisure activities in Taiwan, what types most interest me? City tours? Mountain hiking? Shopping? Night life?

For Big Surgeries, Think Big

If you're heading abroad for a tooth whitening or a new set of dentures, you can skip this. However, if you're going under the knife for major surgery, including

- open-heart surgery of any kind
- any type of transplant
- invasive cancer treatment
- orthopedic surgery
- spinal surgery of any kind

you want to be certain you're getting the best. Your life is at stake. For big surgeries, you should head to the big hospitals that have performed large numbers of *exactly* your kind of procedure, with the accreditation and success ratios to prove it. A JCI-accredited hospital—such as Min-Sheng General Hospital or Taipei Medical University–Wan Fang Hospital—carries the necessary staff, medical talent, administrative infrastructure, expensive instrumentation, and institutional followup needed to pull off a complex larger surgery. They make it look easy. They've done thousands of jobs like yours. It's almost routine. You want that. (**Note:** For more information on the Joint Commission International, see "The What and Why of JCI," below. See also "Alternatives to JCI.")

Be sure to ask about success and morbidity rates *for your particular procedure;* find out how they compare with those in your home country. Finally, ask your surgeon how many surgeries *of exactly your procedure* he or she has performed in the past two years. While there are no set standards, fewer than ten is not so good. More than 50 are much better.

Step 3: Choose a Reliable, Fun Companion

3 This is such an important component of successful health travel that we've dedicated an entire chapter to it, Chapter Six, "For Companions."

Folks who journey to far-flung places for medical treatment fare much better with a companion than if they go solo. Whether a mate or friend or family member, the right companion can provide great help and support before, during, and after treatment. Together, you and your companion may also add in some fun and adventure when your health permits.

Most health travelers choose either a good friend or spouse as a companion. If you have the luxury of choice, make sure the two of you won't be packing a lot of emotional baggage for the trip. The successful medical journey requires large and prolonged doses of support. Ideally, you should get on fabulously with your capable, reliable, organized, and fun companion.

If you've already found a willing and able companion, you are blessed. Be sure to involve him or her in the early planning stages. That's the best way to cement the relationship and learn at the outset if you'll be compatible. Ask your companion to accompany you to your hometown doctor's office, help with second opinions, and make initial international inquiries. You'll begin to work as a team. If you don't feel comfortable at the early stages, find a cordial, diplomatic way to part company.

And always remember to be as supportive and complimentary of your companion as you can possibly be. Your companion is a treasure. Cherish the relationship.

How can you choose the right companion? Three words: Capable. Organized. Fun.

Above all, travel with an individual you can count on in any number of circumstances. From taking notes in your doctor's office to talking your way past a snarly customs agent to fetching a post-surgery prescription, you'll be immeasurably aided and comforted by having someone beside you who will take the job seriously and stay with the program.

Good organizational skills are essential. No job description is complete without that requirement, and the same holds true for your companion. He or she will remind you to bug the travel agency for your passport renewal application, help you organize and email your medical documentation, keep track of your in-country appointments, monitor your prescribed post-treatment regimen, encourage you to follow your doctor's orders, and assist with myriad other tasks that call for sustained bouts of left-brain activity.

Step 4: Find Dr. Right

4 For most folks considering a medical trip abroad, this step is the most challenging — and perhaps the most emotionally charged. If you follow a few basics and caveats, however, you'll find the process far less mysterious and daunting. Remember, the final choice in selecting a physician — as with the decision of whether to travel at all — remains always in your hands.

Here are some tips to aid you in your search:

✦ **Insist on English.** While this advice may sound provincial and harshly xenophobic, if English is your only tongue, then insist that the parties you're working with speak English. Your health is too important to risk important information getting lost in translation.

Don't settle for poor English. Do your best to listen and understand, but if you find yourself constantly asking people to repeat themselves, don't blame yourself. Hospitals and clinics that cater to an international clientele typically have English-speaking staff. If not, then apologize graciously for your lack of language skills, and move on.

✦ **Seek Dr. Right, not Dr. Personality.** Okay, if a practitioner candidate is downright rude to you, then move on, but otherwise, give your physician some "personality latitude," at least initially. Focus on skill sets, credentials, and accreditations, not charm.

Even in this country, many of the finest medical practitioners are technicians. While they may love what they do and be quite good at their chosen specialty, their personal presentation skills may be lacking. This is doubly true where language and cultural differences create additional social awkwardness.

Use your judgment and give the charm factor — or lack of it — the benefit of the doubt. If credentials and other criteria check out, and if you're otherwise comfortable with your choice, then charm and personality can probably take a back seat.

✦ **Expect good service.** Although patience is often required when corresponding with international healthcare providers, rudeness should never be excused, and no culture condones it. If anything, you're likely to encounter greater courtesy and graciousness in Taiwan than in your home country.

In corresponding with hospitals and clinics overseas, you will often find yourself directly in contact with your physician or surgeon. The good news is that you're engaged in a real dialogue with the professional who will be treating you. The downside is that he or she is probably very busy. Expect delays — sometimes two or three days — for return email or phone calls. If it's been longer, then politely but firmly request a response.

Ten "Must-Ask" Questions for Your Physician Candidate

Be sure to make the following initial inquiries of the physician(s) you're interviewing. Note that for some of these questions, there's no right or wrong answer. Your initial round of inquiry will help establish a dialogue. If the doctor is evasive, hurried, or frequently interrupted, or if you can't understand his or her English, then either dig deeper or move on.

1. *What are your credentials? Where did you receive your medical degree? Where was your internship? What types of continuing education workshops have you attended recently?* The right international physician either has credentials posted on the Web or will be happy to email you a complete résumé.

2. *How many patients do you see each month?* Hopefully, more than 50 and less than 500. The physician who says "I don't know" should make you suspicious. Doctors should be in touch with their customer base and have such information readily available.

3. *To what associations do you belong?* Any worthwhile physician or surgeon is a member of at least one medical association. Your practitioner should be keeping good company with others in the field.

4. *How many patients have you treated who have had my condition?* There's safety in numbers, and you'll want to know them. Find out how many general procedures your intended hospital has performed. Ask how many of your specific treatments for your specific condition your candidate doctor has personally conducted. While numbers vary according to procedure, five cases are not good. Fifty or 200 are much better.

5. *What are the fees for your initial consultation?* Answers will vary, and you should compare prices with those of other physicians you interview. Some consultations are free; some are deducted from the bill, should you choose to be treated with that physician; some are a straight nonrefundable fee. In any event, it pays to have this information in advance.

6. *May I call you on your cell phone before, during, and after treatment?* Direct and personal access to a doctor is foreign to many patients' experience. Yet most international physicians stay in close, direct contact with their patients, and cell phones are their tools of choice. When physicians aren't treating patients, you'll find cells or headsets glued to their ears.

7. *What medical and personal health records do you need to assess my condition and treatment needs?* Most physicians require at least the basics: recent notes and recommendations from consultations with your local physician or specialist, x-rays directly related to your condition, perhaps a patient history, and other health records. Be wary of the physician who requires no personal paperwork.

8. *Do you practice alone, or with others in a clinic or hospital?* "Safety in numbers" is a good bet on this front. Look for a physician who practices among a group of certified professionals with a broad range of related skills.

For surgery:

9. *Who's holding the knife during my procedure? Do you do the surgery yourself, or do your assistants do the surgery?* This is one area where delegation isn't desirable. You want specific assurances that all the trouble you went through to find the right surgeon isn't wasted because the procedure will actually be performed by your practitioner's protégé.

10. *Are you the physician who oversees my entire treatment, including pre-surgery, surgery, prescriptions, physical therapy recommendations, and post-surgery checkups?* For more extensive surgical procedures, you want the designated team captain. While that's usually the surgeon, check to make sure.

Step 5: Get to Know Your Hospital or Clinic

5 At this point, you've probably chosen a date and destination for your treatment, settled on one or two physicians you like, and perhaps even scheduled a consultation. Excellent! You've made great headway, and most of the heavy lifting is behind you.

Before you start booking air travel and accommodations or planning the more relaxing parts of the trip, you'll be wise to do some additional sleuthing, beginning with your treatment center. Although detail-driven, this investigation is not as daunting as it sounds, and most of your research involves simple fact-checking. Here's what to do and how:

+ *Check hospital accreditation.* If you're looking into a treatment that requires hospital care, check to see whether the center is JCI-accredited. (See "The What and Why of JCI," below.) While JCI accreditation is not essential, it's an important new benchmark and the only medically oriented seal of approval for international hospitals and clinics. Learning that your treatment center is JCI-approved lends a comfort to your research process, and the remainder of your searching and checking need not be as rigorous. That said, many excellent hospitals, while not JCI-approved, have received local accreditation at the same levels as the world's best treatment centers. (See "Alternatives to JCI," below.)

+ *Check for affiliations and partnerships.* Did you know that many of the best overseas hospitals enjoy close partnerships with universities and medical centers in other countries? For example, Taipei Medical University–Wan Fang Hospital is affiliated with Brigham and Women's Hospital in Boston (US), Nippon Medical School (Japan), National University Hospital (Singapore), and Santa Chiara Hospital (Italy). Chang-Bing Show Chwan Health Care Center Park has relationships with Johns Hopkins University (US), St. Joseph Hospital (Canada), and Oyamada Memorial Hospital (Japan).

✦ *Learn about success rates.* Although smaller clinics don't offer such information, the larger and more established hospitals freely publish their "success rates" or "morbidity rates." These are usually calculated as a ratio of successful operations to overall number of operations performed. For larger surgeries (such as cardiovascular and orthopedic), success rates of 98+ percent are on par with those found in the world's best hospitals. For common surgeries, you should further investigate any rates lower than 98 percent.

> Did you know that many of the best overseas hospitals enjoy close partnerships with universities and medical centers in other countries?

✦ *Learn about number of surgeries.* Most large hospitals will happily furnish information on numbers of surgeries performed. Generally, the more the better, for there's safety in numbers on this front. For example, National Cheng Kung University Hospital in Tainan City performs nearly 1,500 joint replacements annually. You will rest easier on your outbound flight knowing that your destination hospital has performed large numbers of procedures with high success rates.

The What and Why of JCI

When you walk into a hospital or clinic in the US and many other Western countries, chances are good it's accredited, meaning that it's in compliance with standards and "good practices" set by an independent accreditation agency. In the US, by far the largest and most respected accreditation agency is the Joint Commission. The commission casts a wide net of evaluation for hospitals, clinics, home healthcare, ambulatory services, and a host of other healthcare facilities and services throughout the country.

Responding to a global demand for accreditation standards, the Joint Commission launched its international affiliate accreditation agency in 1999, the Joint Commission International (JCI). In order to be accredited by the JCI, an international healthcare provider must meet the same set of rigorous standards set forth in the US by the Joint Commission.

At this writing, 166 hospitals outside the US have been JCI-approved, with more coming on board each month. This is good news for the medical traveler, who can walk with greater confidence into a JCI-accredited facility, knowing standards are high and staff, procedures, instrumentation, and administrative infrastructure are monitored regularly.

Please note that many very fine hospitals and clinics in Taiwan and other countries are not yet JCI-accredited, but they may soon be. If you're considering one of these hospitals, ask questions about accreditation and standards. Gather data until you are satisfied about the quality of both a facility and its care providers.

A general rule of thumb for a global patient, particularly if you're planning on major surgery, is to first seek out JCI-approved sites. Then, when you've settled on a JCI-approved hospital, don't stop there. Rigorously scrutinize your physician's or surgeon's educational background, certification, and affiliations.

JCI's Web site carries far more information than you'll ever want to explore on accreditation standards and procedures. To view a current roster of JCI-accredited hospitals abroad, go to www.jointcommission international.org; in the left column, click "JCI Accredited Organizations."

Alternatives to JCI

When researching hospitals and clinics abroad, you'll often come across the phrase "ISO-accredited." Based in Geneva, Switzerland, the International Organization for Standardization (ISO) is a 157-country network of national standards institutes that approves and accredits a wide range of product and service sectors worldwide, including hospitals and clinics. ISO mostly oversees facilities and administration, *not healthcare procedures, practices, and methods.* Thus, while ISO certification is good to see, it's of limited value in terms of your treatment.

Other organizations around the world set standards and accredit hospitals, and some may be as careful in their procedures protocols as JCI — or not. JCI is the only organization that demands the equivalent of US standards in hospitals accredited abroad. Other organizations that accredit in non-JCI countries include the International Society for Quality in Health Care (ISQua), Australian Council of Healthcare Standards, Canadian Council on Health Services Accreditation, Irish Health Services Accreditation Board, Council for Health Services Accreditation of Southern Africa, Japan Council for Quality in Health Care, and Egyptian Health Care Accreditation Organization. If you are considering a hospital accredited by one of these organizations, it pays to investigate the criteria the organization applies and determine to your own satisfaction that the standards are sufficient and appropriate to your needs.

Step 6: Follow Up with Credentials

6 Once you've located one or two competent physicians, be sure to obtain their résumés. Many physicians post such data on the Web. If your candidates don't, then request that they send you full background information, including education, degrees, areas of specialty, number of years in practice, number of patients served, and association memberships.

✦ **Get references, recommendations, and referrals.** If possible, speak with some of the doctor's former patients to get their feedback. Understandably, many former patients wish their privacy respected, and international law protects us all in that regard. Thus, it's often difficult for a physician to put you in direct contact with a former patient.

If you're unable to talk with former patients, ask your physician to provide you with testimonials, newspaper or magazine articles, and letters of recommendation — in short, anything credible that will help you assess this individual's expertise. If you're using the services of a health travel agency, ask your representative to check credentials and background of physicians to help you narrow your search.

Specifically, here's what you're looking for:

✦ **Education.** What universities and medical schools were attended? What degrees are held and when were they awarded? Has the doctor earned any special achievement awards or honors? Ask your candidate physician or the medical staff to email you a copy of the doctor's résumé or CV if it isn't available online. If you want to take your search a step further, contact the universities, associations, and references listed in the résumé to verify authenticity.

✦ **Certification.** Exactly what is this physician licensed to practice? If you're having a knee replacement done, then you want a certified orthopedic surgeon cutting into your joint.

✦ **Professional history.** How long has he or she been practicing, and where? If a surgeon, how many surgeries have been performed and what types of procedures? Information on presentations, publications, honors, and awards gained along the career path will help you evaluate a doctor's talent, performance, and commitment to his or her trade.

✦ **Affiliations.** With what medical and related associations is the physician affiliated? Information about community involvement is useful as well.

✦ **Continuing education.** Mandatory in many countries, continuing education helps a physician stay abreast of new trends in his or her field. Most good physicians travel at least once a year to accredited conferences and workshops. Find out where your doctor goes and how often.

✦ **Patient references and letters of recommendation.** Nearly as useful as professional histories are reference letters or letters of recommendation from patients, colleagues, or other credible sources.

For more information, see "Ten 'Must-Ask' Questions for Your Physician Candidate," earlier in this chapter.

Step 7: Gather Your Medical Records

7 Once you've established a relationship or scheduled a consultation with one or more overseas physicians, they'll probably ask to see supporting information about your medical needs. Such data usually include the following:

✦ Reports or written recommendations from your local specialist related to your condition

✦ X-rays or imaging reports from your specialist's office or your radiology lab

✦ Test results from your specialist's office or third-party laboratories

Depending upon your treatment, some physicians may ask for additional data, including your general medical history, surgical records, or pathology reports from previous treatments.

Some patients are timid about requesting health information from their doctors. If you're one of those people, it's important for you to know that in the US and many other Western countries, any physician, surgeon, specialist, hospital, or laboratory you visit is *required by law* to provide you with copies of any and all medical information they've compiled about you. These data include consent forms, consultation records, lab reports, test results, x-rays, immunization history, and any other information compiled as a result of your visits. Although most won't require payment for making copies, your doctor or laboratory has the right to charge you a nominal fee for this service.

These days more and more medical information is going digital, particularly all-important x-rays and other imaging data. When you request your medical records, ask staff to email you the data in digital form and provide you with a hard copy as well. If you can obtain only hard-copy documents, then have them scanned.

If you're uncomfortable with technology and computers, perhaps your companion or a friend or family member can tweak the paperwork into the form of an electronic file (scanning is not time-consuming for those who know how). A full-service copy shop or office supply center can convert hard-copy paperwork to digital files for a nominal fee, and you'll save real money on international courier costs if you transmit via email instead. Overseas physicians generally prefer digital records, particularly x-rays, which are easier to study and manipulate in this form.

> Any physician, surgeon, specialist, hospital, or laboratory you visit is *required by law* to provide you with copies of any and all medical information they've compiled about you.

Continuity of Care — Critical to Success

Continuity of care can be a challenge for patients who travel for medical procedures, say Steven Gerst, MD, and John Linss of MedicaView International (www.medicaview.com). Typically, the patient's primary physician diagnoses the condition and then suggests treatment. When the patient chooses to travel to another location or country to receive the treatment, the primary physician is too often left out of the process.

Similarly—and amazingly enough—many traveling patients engage a facility to perform a procedure without speaking directly to the surgeon before arriving. The patient and the hospital's international patient services coordinator may use email for preliminary communications. There may also be a telephone call or two with the coordinator. But the surgeon may not become actively involved until the patient arrives at the facility.

Too many patients make the assumption that a diagnosis is the "end of the story" and that contact with the coordinator is all that is required. *They could not be more wrong!*

Establish Communication!

If you're the patient, insist that you must speak to the surgeon who will perform the procedure *before* you schedule your travel. You may communicate via teleconference, videoconference, or voice over Internet protocol (VOIP).

It is equally important that you establish communication between your primary (hometown) doctor and your in-country surgeon so followup care is prearranged. Because of time and language differences, this advance planning may be difficult, but it is essential. Complications and misunderstandings can arise if your doctors are not communicating properly. For example, after a knee replacement or a kidney transplant, many concerns and complications can arise during the long period of recuperation. Lack of communication can result in unnecessary hardships and potential returns to surgery.

Once you choose to go outside your physician's primary network, few mechanisms currently exist to encourage and facilitate ongoing consultations. *You must establish your own.* Critical information about your case can be lost if you don't. *Be proactive!* Here and abroad, it is usually up to you, the patient, to keep the dialogue going between your physicians.

Persistence is important, and email's effectiveness independent of time zones comes in handy—once you get the doctors in the habit of emailing each other and you. A secure online collaboration tool is even better because it can keep all communications in one place where they are available to all participants at any time.

Have Your Most Current Medical Records

Once you have established contact with an overseas doctor (or surgeon) and facility, provide them with your most current medical records. If you have a chronic condition and you've finally said "enough," your medical records may be a year or more old. If they are, visit your physician to obtain new laboratory tests, x-rays, magnetic resonance imaging (MRI) or computed tomography (CT) scans— whatever your overseas provider needs.

Medical records can be transmitted in two ways: you can send paper copies or disks by postal or courier service, or you can send electronic documents via a secure online service. An online service is preferable for several reasons. First, it gets the records in the hands of the surgeon more quickly. Second, it creates a secure repository that can be accessed by both your physician and your surgeon. Third and most important, digital records create a foundation for aftercare collaboration.

Collaboration Between Your Local Doctor and Your Overseas Surgeon

Transferring your medical records may get your local doctor communicating with your overseas doctor for the first time. This can be achieved though email, telephone, or a private group set-up in an environment specifically designed for that purpose. Often such an environment is part of an online repository system then provides a secure place for collaboration between the doctors via protected blog, chat, email, and VOIP.

The next collaboration between doctors should occur after surgery. The overseas surgeon should notify your physician, preferably through an online system, of the details of the surgery and the aftercare protocol.

Once you return home and are again under the care of your physician, collaboration and consultation should continue. This collaboration should carry on until you are released from care with a clean bill of health.

Complete Documentation

Frequently, when such a repository system is not utilized, patients return home lacking the complete documentation their local physician needs to oversee ongoing care. The absence of information compromises a physician's effectiveness and threatens the patient's health.

Be sure to ask the surgical facility if access is available to an electronic system of medical record-sharing and physician collaboration. If not, request that your overseas healthcare providers subscribe to one to ensure that you can keep your at-home physician informed.

At a minimum, make sure your in-country facility provides you with complete records when you return home. Also make sure you keep your hometown physician involved from the first day. Good continuity of care is essential for a successful outcome.

Remember, as a patient, you need to take responsibility for the quality and consistency of the care you receive. If you don't, no one else will!

Step 8: Plan Your Recuperation and Recovery

8 For patients abroad, the days or weeks you spend post-treatment can be particularly difficult. Perhaps you were on the road vacationing prior to treatment, and now you're ready to head home. Or seemingly urgent work challenges are piling up back at the office. Or you're just feeling far away and becoming homesick.

Any surgeon, dentist, or other medical specialist can tell you that if complications are going to develop, they're most likely to occur in the first few days following treatment. That's the time when your body is doing everything it can to compensate for the stress and trauma of your treatment. Rest and a healthful lifestyle are essential during recovery, but in these busy, overworked times, many people don't take recuperation as seriously as they should. At the first glimmer of normalcy, everyone wants to be off and running again.

Do yourself and your loved ones a big favor: follow your doctor's post-treatment orders, allowing your body and spirit time to return to health. It's not that much more time out of your life. For extensive dental work, recovery is usually a matter of a few days. Even the more invasive surgeries have you back to something approaching normalcy within a few weeks.

You might be surprised—and encouraged—to learn that some hospitals in Taiwan are affiliated with recovery and recuperation accommodations. Serviced apartments and specialty hotels are available in some locations. Services may include

- ✦ **On-site medical staff** to assist with bathing, getting in and out of bed, physical therapy, medication, and more

- ✦ **Gyms** and other accommodations for physical therapy and daily exercise

- ✦ **Room service** for meals and laundry

- ✦ **Internet access**

- ✦ **Liaison with hospitals**

Another big plus for recovery accommodations is the company you keep. The guests are people like you who have recently undergone treatment. There's comfort in sharing experiences, and dinner-table conversations with fellow patients can yield a wealth of medical tips and travel advice. If recovery retreats are not offered in the region of Taiwan you've chosen, ask your hospital contacts for recommendations on hotels or apartments near your treatment facility.

Step 9: Create Your Health Travel Vacation

9 For most health travelers, vacations take a back seat to treatment and recovery. Many simply don't have the time or motivation to tack a vacation onto an already time-consuming health travel trip. Some patients require more invasive procedures with longer recovery times, and the planning alone (not to mention the usual discomforts of recuperation) knocks a fun-filled vacation clean out of the picture.

Medical travelers planning for less demanding treatments, such as light cosmetic surgery or nonsurgical dentistry, should take a brief inventory of their treatment schedule and time requirements. Ask the following questions:

✦ How many appointments does my treatment require?

✦ How long should I remain near my treatment center during my stay?

✦ How long is my expected recuperation period?

Unexpected tests, appointment reshuffles, and travel delays can eat up leisure time. As a rule, the treatment part of your trip will probably be three or four days longer than your appointment schedule indicates.

Whether you can squeeze in a vacation or not, the most important consideration is your health. Focus on your treatment and try not to bite off too much. Remember that you can always take a vacation later, happily spending the money you saved by being treated abroad. And if you find yourself feeling up to a little sightseeing post-procedure, you can usually schedule tours with 24-hours' notice while in-country. This approach allows you to avoid the fees that may be charged should you have to cancel an excursion booked farther in advance.

Step 10: Book Air Travel and Accommodations

10 Why isn't this the first step? Although it may seem counterintuitive to book your travel and accommodations last, remember that once you've decided to go to Taiwan for your treatment, you must first select a treatment center and physician and schedule your consultations or procedure. Only at that point can you begin contacting airlines and hotels; otherwise you're likely to spend needless effort and expense changing itineraries.

You can see now why planning ahead is so important to successful medical travel. Some airlines and most hotels levy stiff penalties for changes and cancellations. That's another reason why it pays to begin your planning 60–90 days prior to your expected departure date and to book your flight *after* you've scheduled your treatment.

When it's time to book air travel and hotels, confirm rates and amenities before pulling out your credit card. First-class and business-class fares are usually quite punishing; they're best paid by jetsetters, corporate executives, and frequent flyers. If you don't mind traveling coach or economy class, you'll save a bundle.

When you're making your travel plans, ask your in-country physician to recommend some hotels near your hospital or treatment center. Some of the larger hospitals in Taiwan have partnerships with hotels for discounted rates. Such information is often posted on their Web sites.

Just Ask

When it comes to asking for special assistance from the airlines, many travelers believe they must be severely handicapped to request a wheelchair or some other service. And some folks are just shy about asking for help or embarrassed to be wheeled around airport corridors and jetways.

Get over it! If you're heading to Taiwan for hip surgery and you've been in chronic pain for three years, there's no shame in requesting a wheelchair, and every airline we contacted ministers happily to medical travelers. In the same vein, if you're still feeling the effects of surgery on your homebound trip, it's perfectly reasonable to request wheelchair assistance.

Airlines ask that you or your companion call to request a wheelchair 48 hours prior to your flight. Then, when you arrive at the airport, check in with the skycap at curbside, where a wheelchair is usually nearby. Remember to tip folks a few dollars for assisting you; they'll appreciate the gesture and remember you the next time your paths cross.

Step 11: Triple-Check Details and Documents

11 In addition to ensuring that the kids, dog, and other loved ones are looked after in your absence, it's crucial on a medical trip to remember to take everything that you and your companion will need. Unlike forgetting your favorite tie or blouse, leaving important documents behind can create unnecessary hassles on the other side of the world.

Make sure you have all your paperwork in order, including travel itinerary, airline tickets or etickets, passports, visas, immunization records, and plenty of cash for airport taxes and any unexpected expenses. Be sure to pack all medical records, consultation notes, agreements, and hard copies of email correspondence. Also remember to take the telephone numbers, fax numbers, and email addresses of all your at-home and in-country contacts.

Pack Smart

You've likely heard the cardinal rule of international travel: pack light. Less to carry means less to lose. Don't worry if you leave behind some basic item, such as shampoo or a comb. Once abroad you can always buy essentials you may have forgotten, and picking up socks or toothpaste is a great excuse for you or your companion to hit the local market.

That said, below are several items you absolutely, positively shouldn't forget:

- Passport
- Visa (if required; upon entry into Taiwan, a 30-day visa is given upon arrival to citizens from many countries; check with your home country's visa office to see if you need one)
- Travel itinerary
- Airline tickets or eticket confirmations
- Driver's license or valid picture ID (in addition to passport)
- Health insurance card or policy
- Enough cash for airport fees and local transportation upon arrival
- Credit card(s)
- ATM card or traveler's checks
- Immunization record
- Hard copies of all appointment schedules and financial agreements
- Prescription medications you're taking and copies of written prescriptions
- Hard-to-find over-the-counter drugs you're taking
- Alcohol-based hand-sanitizing gel (for cleaning hands while traveling)
- Your medical records, current x-rays, consultation reports, and notes
- Phone numbers, postal addresses, and email addresses of people you need or want to contact at home or in-country
- Travel journal for notes, expense records, and receipts

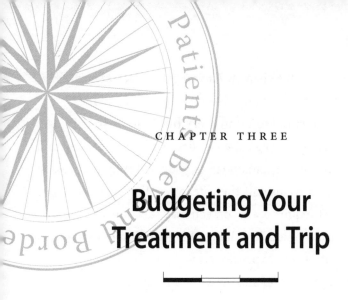

CHAPTER THREE

Budgeting Your Treatment and Trip

First Things First: Consider Your Treatment and Travel Preferences

As with any other trip, your health travel costs will depend largely upon your tastes, lifestyle preferences, length of stay, side trips, and pocketbook. A patient flying first-class on Cathay Pacific Airways and staying at the luxurious Les Suites Ching-Cheng Hotel in Taipei can naturally expect fewer savings than one who spends frequent-flyer miles and lodges in a nearby — and perfectly satisfactory — international tourist-class hotel.

To set reasonable expectations and avoid surprises, you should calculate an estimate of your trip's cost. This chapter offers advice, tips, and milestones that will help you with your financial planning.

To derive an estimate of your health travel costs and savings, we suggest you use the "*Patients Beyond Borders* Budget Planner" at the end of this chapter. As you get an idea of each separate cost, a realistic estimate of your savings will emerge.

Don't feel pressured to fill in every line item in your Budget Planner. Focus on the big expenses first, such as treatment and airfare, and fill in the remainder as your planning progresses. You probably won't use all the categories. For example, some countries don't require a visa; or, you may stay only at a hospital and never visit a hotel. The Budget Planner simply lists all the common health travel expenses. As you plan, you can fill in the blanks that apply to you and arrive at a rough estimate of your total costs — and your savings!

As you complete the items in your Budget Planner, consider the following:

Passport and Visa

US citizens who don't have a passport and are purchasing one for the first time should budget around US$200 for fees, photographs, and shipping. Renewal of a passport in the US costs about US$150. Fees in other countries vary widely; check with the appropriate government office.

Visa requirements vary widely by country, too. Upon entry into Taiwan, most visitors receive a 30-day visa. Health travelers can arrange for longer stays if necessary. As of this writing, visas for Taiwan cost about US$66 for a single entry and US$132 for multiple entries. The visa application fee for US citizens is US$131. Citizens from some other countries can obtain visas without charge.

To avoid punishing rush charges and needless pre-treatment

anxiety, take care of your passport and visa purchases early — passports at least two months in advance of your trip.

Airfare

Air transportation will likely be your biggest nontreatment cost. It pays to shop hard for bargains. If you're okay flying coach, by all means do so; business- and first-class international travel are wildly expensive.

If you have a *trusted* travel agency, use it, although with caution. Most have side deals with airlines, and their commissions and fees can cut into your savings.

If you're comfortable using the Internet, take advantage of one of the many discount online travel agencies, such as Orbitz (www.orbitz.com), Expedia (www.expedia.com), Travelocity (www.travelocity.com), or CheapTickets (www.cheaptickets .com). Or go to individual airlines' Web sites, where you can sometimes snag special Internet fares.

Auction and deep-discount services, such as Priceline (www .priceline.com), take a little more knowledge and patience. Exercise buyer caution with some of the lesser-known "cheap-trip" agencies.

> Air transportation will likely be your biggest nontreatment cost. It pays to shop hard for bargains.

Action Item: **Keep your budget current. As your plans change, so will your cost estimate.**

International Entry and Exit Fees

For Taiwan, entry and exit fees are usually included in the airline ticket. The fee is about US$10 per person. Proof of payment must be retained for checking by airport officials upon departure.

Rental Car

When traveling, some people feel they can't manage without a car. Yet international car rentals are expensive, big-city parking is a hassle, and driving in a foreign country can land you in the hospital well ahead of your scheduled stay. Even the most adventurous health traveler should think twice about driving a car while full of sutures and post-operative medications.

It's better to use taxis or limousines. They're comparatively inexpensive and, despite the overworked horror stories, cab drivers are generally cooperative when you follow the basics found in any travel guide.

As a medical traveler, your transportation needs — at least immediately pre- and post-treatment — are likely to be limited to hotels and restaurants. Your hospital or hotel usually provides local transportation free or at modest cost.

If you're planning to head out of town on a post-treatment jaunt, then renting a car is fine. Just be sure that you or your companion books the car in advance, as sometimes a conference, festival, or other special event can deplete rental inventories fast.

Other Transportation

Transportation to and from the airport will probably be handled by the hospital or the hotel where you or your companion will reside. You should budget for the cost of transportation to and from your at-home airport, as well as for in-country transportation costs. Buses, taxis, and trains are everywhere in Taiwan; they are cheap, convenient, and efficient. US$200 should cover nearly any two-week trip.

Companions

Most health travelers we interviewed were glad that a friend or family member accompanied them. In addition to providing love, support, and a shoulder to cry on during difficult moments, companions can attend to myriad details. Many of those who traveled alone wished they'd had a companion or assistant during those inevitable trying times even the healthiest of tourists experience.

You should budget for the additional airfare and meals for your companion and — depending on whether you'll be doubling up — lodging. Items you can usually share include local taxi rides, mobile phone, and computer and Internet services. Items you can't share include passport and visa costs, airfare, airport fees and taxes, rail fares, meals, and entertainment.

Treatment

Treatment costs vary widely, depending upon the procedure, preferred country, room choice, service options, and post-treatment care.

When you are evaluating a treatment center or physician candidate, request the cost details in writing (email is okay), including the prices for basic treatment plus ancillaries, such as anesthesia, room fees, prescribed medications, nursing services, and more. Other useful questions include these: Are meals included in my hospital stay? Do you supply a bed for my companion? Is there an Internet connection in the room or lobby?

Then, once you've decided where you're going, check, double-check, confirm, and reconfirm your hospital's and physician's quotes.

Lodging During Treatment

These costs are straightforward and are largely a function of your tastes and pocketbook. If you're not staying in a hospital or treatment center, search for a hotel or serviced apartment near the hospital. Long cross-town treks can be time-consuming, hot, frenzied, and costly. Your doctor or your treatment center's staff can provide you with a list of preferred hotels nearby.

Post-Treatment Lodging

Unless you're undergoing nothing more than tests or light dental work, it's a good idea to stick around for at least a week post-treatment instead of jumping on the first plane out. Your physician will want to keep an eye on how your recovery is progressing. We highly recommend you take advantage of this important period to gain strength, guard against complications, and adjust to new medications, physical therapies, and lifestyle changes.

Several hospitals in Taiwan offer nearby serviced apartments or other recovery facilities, which may include resident nurses and other staff who can assist you with your post-treatment needs. Such facilities are modern, comfortable, and convenient, and your stay there can be the most relaxing part of your trip. Ask your treatment center about any such facilities in the region. Whether you're recuperating in a serviced apartment or hotel, budget at least US$150 – US$300 per day for lodging, meals, and post-treatment services.

> Your doctor or your treatment center's staff can provide you with a list of preferred hotels nearby.

Meals

If you're staying in a hospital, most of your meals will probably be provided, and the food is often surprisingly good. Many hospitals in Taiwan offer reasonable meal plans for companions. Ask the facility or your physician's staff about costs for hospital meals. Otherwise, budget your dining out according to taste, both for you and for your companion. Any reputable travel guide to Taiwan can give you a good idea about restaurant costs. And of course, avoid street food and restaurants of questionable repute. You don't want to complicate your medical travels with a rising bout of indigestion (or worse) just prior to your treatment.

Tips

Tipping is not usually expected in Taiwan, usually because most hotels and restaurants add a 10 percent service charge to the bill. In places where the service charge is not included, visitors may want to leave a small gratuity for service personnel. Tipping is always optional, but a small amount for bell service or valet parking is usually a good idea.

Leisure Travel

Many health travelers plan a vacation for either before or after treatment. While this expense isn't strictly a part of your health travel, you may want to add the costs of vacation-related lodging, transportation, meals, and other expenses into your estimated budget.

The $6,000 Rule Revisited

We've mentioned it elsewhere in this book, but it's worth stating again: A good monetary barometer of whether your medical trip is financially worthwhile is the *Patients Beyond Borders* "$6,000 Rule." If your total quote for hometown treatment (including consultations, procedure, and hospital stay) is US$6,000 or more, you'll probably save money traveling abroad for your care. If it's less than US$6,000, you're likely better off having your treatment at home.

The application of this rule varies, of course, depending on your financial position and lifestyle preferences. For some, a savings of US$500 might offset the hassles of travel. For others who might be traveling anyway, savings considerations are fuzzier.

Patients Beyond Borders Budget Planner

Item	Cost	Comment
IN-COUNTRY		
Passport/Visa	$200.00	For passport and visa, non-expedited
Rush charges, if any:		
Treatment Estimate		
Procedure:		
Hospital room, if extra:		Often included in treatment package
Lab work, x-rays, etc.:		
Additional consultations:		
Tips/gifts for staff:	$100.00	
Other:		
Other:		
Post-Treatment		
Recuperation lodging:		Hospital room or hotel
Physical therapy:		
Prescriptions:		
Concierge services:		Optional
Other:		
Other:		
Airfare		
You:		
Your companion:		
Other travelers:		
Airport exit fee:	$25.00	
Other:		
Other:		
In-Country Transportation		
Taxis, buses, limos:	$100.00	
Rental car:		
Other:		
Other:		

Patients Beyond Borders Budget Planner (*continued*)

Item	Cost	Comment
Room and Board		
Hotel:		
Food:		
Entertainment/sightseeing:		
Transportation:		
Other:		
Other:		
"While You're Away" Costs		
Pet sitter/house sitter:		
Other:		
Other:		
IN-COUNTRY TREATMENT SUBTOTAL		
HOMETOWN		
Procedure:		
Lab work, x-rays, etc.:		
Hospital room, if extra:		
Additional consultations:		
Physical therapy:		
Prescriptions:		
Other:		
Other:		
HOMETOWN SUBTOTAL		
TOTAL SAVINGS:		Subtract "In-Country" Subtotal from "Hometown" Subtotal

Patients Beyond Borders Sample Budget Planner

Item	Cost	Comment
IN-COUNTRY		
Passport/Visa	$200.00	For passport and visa, non-expedited
Rush charges, if any:		
Treatment Estimate		
Procedure:	$9,000.00	
Hospital room, if extra:		Often included in treatment package
Lab work, x-rays, etc.:	$45.00	
Additional consultations:	$200.00	
Tips/gifts for staff:	$100.00	
Other:		
Other:		
Post-Treatment		
Recuperation lodging:	$1,100.00	Hospital room or hotel
Physical therapy:		
Prescriptions:	$65.00	
Concierge services:	$300.00	Optional
Other:		
Other:		
Airfare		
You:	$880.00	
Your companion:	$880.00	
Other travelers:		
Airport exit fee:	$25.00	
Other:		
Other:		
In-Country Transportation		
Taxis, buses, limos:	$100.00	
Rental car:		
Other:		
Other:		

Patients Beyond Borders Sample Budget Planner (*continued*)

Item	Cost	Comment
Room and Board		
Hotel:	$1,500.00	
Food:	$650.00	
Entertainment/sightseeing:	$500.00	
Transportation:		
Other:		
Other:		
"While You're Away" Costs		
Pet sitter/house sitter:	$300.00	
Other:		
Other:		
IN-COUNTRY SUBTOTAL	$15,845.00	
HOMETOWN		
Procedure:	$55,000.00	
Lab work, x-rays, etc.:	$375.00	
Hospital room, if extra:	$4,400.00	
Additional consultations:		
Physical therapy:	$400.00	
Prescriptions:	$500.00	
Other:		
Other:		
HOMETOWN SUBTOTAL	$60,675.00	
TOTAL SAVINGS:	$44,830.00	Subtract "In-Country" Subtotal
		from "Hometown" Subtotal

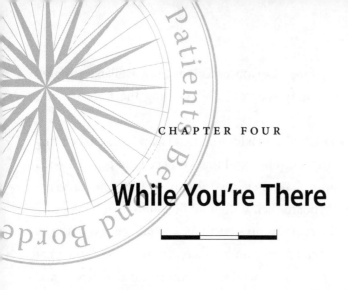

While You're There

First Things First: Arm Yourself with Information

Now that you have settled on a treatment facility, made appointments with one or more physicians, booked your airfare and hotel, and arranged transportation, the hard part is behind you — except, of course, for the treatment itself. You'll find that once you arrive in-country, you will be greeted graciously, with help and support from hotel and hospital staff and sometimes even a friendly bystander.

But before you embark on an airplane journey overseas, you should read, ask questions, and learn as much as you can about your destination. *Patients Beyond Borders: Taiwan Edition* can't begin to provide all the important information you need about international travel — or even all the specifics about Taiwan. Yet we do want to point you to a few important basics to get you started. Everything else you need is readily available through a number of handy sources. (See "Getting the Information," below.)

If you've not done much international travel prior to booking your health trip, keep in mind that you need not be a seasoned travel veteran to have a successful trip. In fact, most international tourists board their outbound flight in blissful ignorance of their destination's culture, customs, and language — and they do just fine. Armed with multiple credit cards, they rent a car or hire a limousine at the airport and head for a beach resort, without giving a thought to the country they're visiting. Many scarcely speak to a native, except perhaps to mumble a few words during shopping sprees or dining out.

> Knowing a little something about the culture, history, geography, and language of your host country will buy you boatloads of goodwill and appreciation.

Health travel is different because you have to be far more concerned about practical matters. Getting things done cooperatively and efficiently will help you and your companion preserve your physical *and* mental health. And most health travelers are interested in saving money when it's prudent to do so.

By pre-arrangement, you'll be interacting closely with local physicians, staff, nurses, and others who live and work in Taiwan. Thus, knowing a little something about the culture, history, geography, and language of the country will buy you boatloads of goodwill and appreciation. A small investment of time and effort in learning something about Taiwan will help you make the right choices and become more confident and proficient when you arrive in-country.

Getting the Information

Travel guides. You've probably seen at least one edition of *Lonely Planet, Insiders' Guide, Frommer's, Fodor's,* or some of the other popular travel series. A host of travel guides has been published for Taiwan. Most of the general information (e.g., history, currency, banking, and transportation) is essentially the same in all the books. *Lonely Planet* guides are generally written for a younger crowd, with information for backpackers as well as five-star travelers. *Frommer's* guides are aimed at an older audience, but like *Lonely Planet, Frommer's* is budget conscious, although somewhat stodgier then its hip counterpart.

It's a good idea to thumb through the pages of various guides in your local bookstore or library and choose the format and presentation that best fits your tastes. Avoid titles such as *Rough Guide . . .* and *Off the Beaten Path. . . .* Save them for your dream adventure vacation.

Since books are not cheap, you might want to head to your local library to borrow three or four titles on Taiwan. Or search the Amazon customer reviews, which offer individual readers' surprisingly erudite, accurate assessments of a book's strengths and shortcomings; then purchase the one or two that sound best.

Be sure to take at least one travel book with you on the trip — it will become your travel bible, filled with notes, dog-eared pages, business cards, phone numbers, email addresses, and random scribblings. Of course, if you're planning a side trip or vacation, you might want a travel guide for those destinations as well. However, if you are a real lover of books, you may be wise to curb your enthusiasm. Books are heavy to carry, and they seem to grow more so the farther you travel.

Maps. While most travel guides contain country and city maps, they are often difficult to read. The print is small and the maps lack detail. If you want or need to know your exact location or if you are planning side trips, a small investment in an oversized street map or road map will yield a large return.

When in-country, bookstores are usually your best bets for high-quality maps and road atlases, but they can be difficult to find, and sellers are frequently out of stock. For that reason, it's often a good idea to buy a map before you travel. Some passport and visa services sell maps at a reasonable price (check online for various services). Amazon has a good supply; just go to www .amazon.com and search for **<city> map** or **<country> map**.

Action Item: Buy a travel guide — and read it!

General Guidelines and Cautions

Here are a few general travel tips and guidelines that will help get you started.

Safety and security. The overriding concern of most patients new to global health travel is safety. That's understandable. In the past five years, this old world has seen several terrorist plots at UK airports (a frequent medical tourist stopover), a military coup in Bangkok (one of the most-traveled medical tourist destinations), peoples' rebellions in Oaxaca and Mexico City (popular with dental travelers), rioting in Budapest (a popular dental and cosmetic surgery destination), and never-ending strife in Israel (an important destination for reproductive and infertility procedures) — to mention only a few.

Obviously, we live in a troubled world. Yet this fact remains: of the more than 3 million patients who traveled for medical treatment in the last five years, not one has died as a result of violence or hostility. As you read this chapter, you'll learn that most health travelers are quite sheltered. Typically, they're chauffeured from the airport to the hospital or hotel, personally driven to consultations, given their meals in their rooms, and chauffeured back to the airport when it's time to go home. All with good reason, as the

> As a medical traveler, you'll be too busy achieving your health goals to be booking risky nights out on the town, hazardous wilderness tours, or adventurous side trips of uncertain outcome.

primary purpose of health travel is to undergo medical treatment. As a medical traveler, you'll be too busy achieving your health goals to be booking risky nights out on the town, hazardous wilderness tours, or adventurous side trips of uncertain outcome.

Crime. Although Taiwan is considered a medium-risk location for crime, the overall violent crime rate in Taiwan remains relatively low. Travelers should avoid certain types of business establishments, such as massage parlors, illegal "barbershops," and illegal "nightclubs," because many of these establishments are run by criminals and located in high-crime areas. In contrast to their counterparts, legal barbershops prominently display the usual grooming services. Illegal nightclubs have no advertisement and are publicized by word of mouth only.

Penalties for breaking the law can be more severe in Taiwan than for similar offenses in Western countries. Persons violating Taiwan's laws, even unknowingly, may be expelled, arrested, or imprisoned. Penalties for illegal drug possession, use, or trafficking in Taiwan are severe, and convicted offenders can expect long jail sentences and heavy fines. Engaging in illicit sexual conduct with children or using or disseminating child pornography in a foreign state is a crime, prosecutable in the traveler's home country.

In Taiwan, counterfeit and pirated goods are widely available. Transactions involving such products may be illegal under local law. In addition, taking them home may result in forfeitures or fines. Travelers are urged to purchase only legally manufactured and sold goods from reputable, established merchants.

Traffic and transportation. Roads in Taiwan's major cities are generally congested, and the many scooters and motorcycles that weave in and out of traffic make driving conditions worse. Pedestrians should exercise caution when crossing streets because many drivers do not respect the pedestrian's right of way. Special caution should be taken when driving on mountain roads, which are typically narrow, winding, and poorly banked, and which may be impassable after heavy rains.

Public transportation, including the buses and high-speed rail, is generally safe in Taiwan, but women should exercise caution when traveling alone in taxis late at night. In several parts of Taiwan, incidents of purse snatching by thieves on motorcycles have been reported.

Aviation safety. The US Federal Aviation Administration (FAA) has assessed Taiwan's Civil Aeronautics Administration (CAA) as being in compliance with International Civil Aviation Organization (ICAO) safety standards for oversight of Taiwan's air carrier operations.

Arrival screening process. The interest of Taiwan's Department of Health (DOH) in early detection and prevention of communicable diseases requires all arriving passengers to have their body temperatures scanned with an infrared thermal apparatus. Only passengers showing symptoms are required by airport personnel to fill out the Communicable Disease Survey Form. Depending on the severity of the symptoms and travel history, certain individuals may then be required to give an on-site specimen or to follow up with local health authorities.

Disaster preparedness. Taiwan is subject to strong earthquakes that can occur anywhere on the island. Taiwan is also hit by typhoons, usually from July to October. Travelers planning a trip to Taiwan can obtain general information about natural disaster preparedness on the Internet from the US Federal Emergency Management Agency (FEMA) at www.fema.gov. The Central Weather Bureau of Taiwan also maintains a Web site that provides information about typhoons and earthquakes at www.cwb.gov.tw.

More safety information. For the latest security information, Americans traveling abroad can monitor the US State Department's Web site at http://travel.state.gov, where the current Worldwide Cautions, Travel Warnings, and Travel Alerts can be found. Up-to-date information on security can also be obtained by calling 1 888 407.4747 toll-free in the US and Canada. Callers outside the US and Canada should use the regular toll line at 1 202 501.4444. These numbers are in operation from 0800 to 2000 hours Eastern Standard Time, Monday through Friday (except US federal holidays).

Currency, credit cards, and banking. Much has changed in our new era of electronic banking, and currency is no exception. Check your local travel guides for specifics. Check with your hospital beforehand to determine accepted forms of payment.

✦ *Cash.* Despite the US dollar's slide, good old American greenbacks — albeit devalued — are usually the best way to get the most for your money, without all the surcharges and hassles that come with traveler's checks and credit cards. If you want to take cold hard cash to cover your entire trip and treatment, be sure that you are confident about carrying that much money. Check with your hotel staff or hospital administration beforehand to determine whether they offer room or lobby safes.

Visitors who wish to carry more than US$10,000 into Taiwan must inform the Directorate General of Customs, Ministry of Finance.

✦ **Traveler's checks.** These somewhat outdated instruments are still accepted by most hotels, hospitals, and restaurants — but usually only for a fee. Be sure to check first with your treatment center on the types of traveler's checks accepted.

✦ **Credit cards.** As convenient as they are, credit cards may not always be your best method of payment, particularly for large transactions (such as settling your hospital bills). Some establishments tack on service charges that can run as high as 10 percent — negating the value of any frequent-flyer miles you might want to earn. Then, adding insult to injury upon your return, your bank statement may reflect an additional 2–5 percent on each transaction. If possible, avoid using your credit card for cash advances, as banks charge big commissions on those. Check with your bank or credit card company before you leave home about its policies concerning international transactions.

✦ **ATMs.** Popping up on nearly every overseas street corner are the ubiquitous ATMs now so indispensable to travelers.

ATMs usually offer exchange rates equal or close to the day's official rate. Prior to your trip, check with your bank on its ATM surcharges, if any.

✦ **International wire transfers.** Avoid them. They are prone to frustrating, bungled attempts at one end or the other. Also avoid black markets and moneychangers.

✦ **Hotel safes.** Most of the hotels and hospitals recommended in this book offer personal safes where you can stash your cash, passports, airline tickets, and other important belongings. Just remember to clean out your safe as you pack for departure! One health traveler reported getting to the airport still woozy on painkillers, fumbling for tickets and money, and becoming hysterical before realizing he had forgotten to empty his safe. He made the plane, a little poorer and a little more gray-haired, after a hectic taxi ride back to the hotel.

When traveling on your own — as you might when shopping for gifts — be sure to take lots of small bills or coins. You don't want to be seen on the streets sorting through a pile of large bills, and most shopkeepers can't or won't break them, leaving you standing there while they trot next door for change. Yet large bills are what you usually get from ATMs, banks, and money exchange offices. Ask for smaller denominations. Your hotel desk or hospital cashier can break big bills. Keep a change purse, and keep it full!

Water. The last thing you need as a patient — pre- or post-treatment — is a case of nausea or diarrhea. Whenever you are traveling, it's a good idea to request bottled water. Check to ensure that the cap's seal is unbroken.

Food. One of the most oft-heard comments from "on the road" patients is about the food. Surprisingly, the complaint isn't about the quality of the hospital meals. Indeed, the heart of the problem is that institutional meals abroad tend to be *too* robust, particularly post-treatment. Patients just out of surgery, who are taking antibiotics, painkillers, and other pharmaceuticals, should not be sampling exotic new taste delights. Until you are well on your way to recovery, ask your hospital dietician for the blandest food possible, and pass the tray of spicy tofu to your companion!

Outside the hospital, avoid "greasy spoons" and street vendors. While veteran travelers and locals have no trouble with street food, the digestive systems of health travelers are not primed to withstand the flora that often thrives in native dishes. The better restaurants and best hotels are safer places to eat, but even there, it's best to choose familiar, bland, fully cooked foods.

Note for women: Make sure you take a scarf to Taiwan. There may be times when you are expected to cover your head.

Dress. If you're staying in a hospital, comfort is your first priority, and your gown will be about as elegant a fashion statement as you'll make. Once on the outside, you should respect local customs for dress. As a nearly universal rule, shorts are frowned upon except at the beach. And shirtless men are almost never seen in town, even on the hottest days. When walking the city, check out what the folks on the streets are wearing; if you're comparably dressed, you'll be fine.

Note for women: Make sure you take a scarf to Taiwan. There may be times when you are expected to cover your head. Also, sleeveless garments, tank tops, camisoles, and micro-mini-skirts are frowned on. Cover your arms and legs in Taiwan.

Getting around town. Ground transportation varies depending upon your destination — from rickshaws and bicycles to motorcycles, buses, and stretch limousines. Generally, your best bet is a good old-fashioned motorized sedan taxi. They come in different shapes and sizes and are usually reliable. Be sure you use only authorized, licensed, or certified taxis. Your hotel concierge can give you specific information on finding the right services at the right price. Make sure the driver understands your destination; if not, find a driver who does. Carry the address and phone number of your hotel, hospital, or recovery apartment with you at all times so you can show your driver where you need to go or phone your hotel if necessary. You needn't tip taxi drivers in Taiwan.

Operator, Information: Staying in Touch While on the Road

When in-country, most folks want to communicate with friends, family, and coworkers back home, and good communications with your caregivers and other medical staff are essential during your stay.

Gone are the days of postcards and telefax, now largely replaced by email, cell phones, Instant Messaging, and other helpful tools. If you're already using email and cell phones at home, you'll no doubt be comfortable in-country once you learn a few new ways of doing things.

Email. The most hassle-free and least expensive way to keep current with loved ones and coworkers is via email. Taiwan offers widespread and excellent Internet access, either free or very cheap. If you take your laptop, avoid traditional dial-up and modem connections. Dialing out from far-flung places can often be more trouble than it's worth, and high-speed access is available nearly everywhere you're likely to visit.

Before leaving on your trip, ask your email or Internet service provider how to log onto your email account using the Web. Follow their instructions to access your email account on the Web and note your username and password, which may be different from those you ordinarily use. If you can't access your email using a Web browser (such as Internet Explorer or Mozilla), consider setting up a temporary email account with one of the many free Web-based services. The three most popular are Hotmail (www.hotmail.com), Yahoo (www.yahoo.com), and Google (www.gmail.com). You can easily cancel the account after you return home.

You'll have no trouble finding Internet access in Taiwan. Most hotels now offer high-speed wireless or Ethernet connections, either in your room or in the lobby. If you choose not to take a

> If you take your laptop, avoid traditional dial-up and modem connections. Dialing out from far-flung places can often be more trouble than it's worth, and high-speed access is available nearly everywhere you're likely to visit.

laptop, many hotels have terminals in their lobbies with Internet connectivity, but the price is often high and the wait may be long. It's usually cheaper and easier to find an Internet café on the street, if you're healthy enough to venture out.

Internet cafés. These abound in Taiwan. They're usually inexpensive, with reliable, fast connections. Internet cafés can be a welcome change of scene from your hotel or treatment center, and they'll sometimes afford you an opportunity to meet and chat with fellow travelers. Your hotel or treatment center staff can tell you where the nearest Internet café is located. Or, you can do a Google search by entering the search terms **<internet café> <city> <Taiwan>.** Expect to pay US$2 – US$6 per hour in an Internet café, with modest extra charges for printing.

The more advanced or adventurous computer user can also deploy a wide range of telecommunications services, including voice over Internet protocol (VOIP), Instant Messenger, Web video chat, and more.

Mobile phones. If you want to hear your loved ones' voices from afar, do a little research into the country you'll be visiting before you leave home. International telecommunications standards vary, as do costs and quality of service. (For more about phone service in Taiwan, see Part Three.) Your best bets may be purchasing or renting a "GSM-enabled" phone, buying an international calling card, or both.

The right mobile phone can be a great travel companion and medical assistant. Not only does a mobile phone allow you to circumvent the hassles of international telephone calling cards, it's usually the way overseas physicians and other caregivers prefer to communicate with their patients. Thus, your in-country calls are likely to be as important as calls to people back home, making a cell phone nearly essential during your stay.

But before you invest in an international mobile phone, check with your hospital. They sometimes offer a mobile phone as part of their service package, and it's much easier to use a phone that's provided for you than to go through the hassle of do-it-yourself.

If a phone is not provided for you, you may want to purchase or rent a "GSM-enabled" phone, along with a prepaid SIM card. Before you do, however, check the cell phone you already own; if it's less than a year old, chances are it is GSM-enabled. Contact your mobile phone service provider to find out if your phone is GSM-enabled. If it is, ask to have it "unlocked." Insist if necessary. Unlocking your phone will allow you to use it much less expensively in any other country.

If you do not have a GSM-enabled phone and your stay abroad will be a month or less, we suggest you buy an inexpensive, unlocked GSM phone. They are now available for less than US$100, along with a prepaid SIM card. That way, you can give your cell phone number to friends and loved ones *before* you leave. Although buying a phone is more expensive than other options, you can circumvent numerous hassles and the dauntingly steep learning curve that goes along with mastering the public pay phone system in many countries overseas. Also, purchasing a GSM-enabled phone is still cheaper than dialing from your hotel room, calling collect, or using a credit card.

Here are a few additional tips for using mobile phones internationally:

✦ Don't let your local mobile phone service talk you into using their GSM plan, which may well be expensive, without allowing you to make in-country, local calls to your physician and other caregivers easily.

✦ If you purchase a GSM phone abroad, be careful about signing up for a plan that might commit you to a year or more of service. Before you pull out your credit card, read the fine print.

✦ If you decide to rent a GSM phone, either at home or in Taiwan, you'll probably be tied into the rental company's calling plan, which can sometimes prove significantly more expensive — even for local, in-country calling. As a rule, if you plan to use your international phone *only* for emergencies, renting may be prudent. Otherwise, purchase a phone; it will come in handy on your next trip abroad!

✦ Even if you can't use your normal cell phone abroad, pack it anyway. Many folks find that upon returning, a cell phone is useful in communicating from the airport or on the way home. Make sure to switch it off before packing so the battery doesn't lose its charge.

International calling cards. If you've ever used international calling cards, you know there's a large and often bewildering array of options, with pros and cons for each.

If you choose to purchase a calling card in-country, chances are you'll be buying a card that you "swipe" through a pay phone, much as you swipe a credit card at your local grocery store. You'll be asked for your authorization code, and after giving it, you can input the phone number. Other calling cards ask you to input a local toll-free phone number and then enter your access code. While these cards are more versatile, you're faced with a whole lot of numbers.

A newer alternative to purchasing calling cards in-country is to sign up on the Internet for an international calling card service, prior to departing. After you register, calling card access information and a PIN code are emailed to you. You can also check your billing status online, add credit to your account, and utilize a host of other services. A simple Web search of **<telephone calling cards>** will bring up dozens of such companies.

If you're having no success with calling cards, remember that you can always head to a pay phone, access the international operator, and call collect. While that's a much more expensive option, you'll at least get through. Or as a last resort, you can call from your hotel room. It's extremely expensive, but it gets the job done. Just remember to keep calls from your room brief.

Additional tips for using telephones abroad:

+ If you want to place international calls directly from your hotel room or use the phone line to dial out on your computer, inquire about the rates before you connect. You'll pay a high premium for such services, and you don't want your phone charges to total more than your room bill!

+ Never call from a pay phone or other calling center that takes Visa or MasterCard without first checking the rates. They're usually rip-offs (including Verizon and other big names), and charges of US$3 – US$5 per minute are common.

✦ When using an international calling card from a payphone, try to find a quiet place and avoid calling from the street, particularly if you are hard of hearing or use a hearing aid. Hotel lobbies are usually quieter.

✦ Many Internet cafés offer reasonably priced international telephone service, a great alternative to calling cards.

Communicating with Your In-Country Caregivers

Voice. Most folks who travel abroad for treatment are stunned to find that physicians and surgeons are generally far more easily accessible than are their doctors back home. When you're in-country, your doctor's preferred method of communication may be the cell phone, which can be used for voice, voice messaging, and text messaging.

As part of your early planning and screening for the right doctor, be sure to ask for his or her cell phone number and ask if it's okay to call with questions or concerns. If it's not okay, then ask how the doctor prefers to stay in touch; ask also for the names and contact information of key staff members. While email is great during the early planning stages, once in-country you'll want to be assured of immediate direct contact and prompt responses to your queries.

Remember that while caregivers abroad are generally friendly and accessible, they are nonetheless quite busy. Keep your phone conversations concise and have a good idea of what you want to say before you call.

Text messaging. Knowing how to use text messaging on your mobile phone is a real plus when communicating with your caregivers. In brief, text messaging is email for mobile phones. It's more widely used abroad than traditional email. Keep your text messages concise, e.g., "Doctor Chang, please call me back soon. I have a problem."

Going under the Knife? Pre- and Post-Surgery Tips and Cautions

Be informed about general and specific pre-treatment precautions. If your physician has not already briefed you (usually in writing), be sure to ask about food, alcohol, pharmaceuticals, and physical activities that may not be allowed prior to surgery. Ask also about the aftercare regimen you will need to follow. Although all surgeries come with the same general precautions, take the time to learn the instructions *specific to your treatment.*

Get There Good to Go

Did you know that patients planning to undergo LASIK eye treatment must not wear contacts for two weeks prior to the operation? Imagine disembarking from a 23-hour trip to Taipei, walking into your doctor's office for your initial consultation wearing contacts, and hearing that for the first time!

The point is this: take the time to learn about the dos and don'ts for your procedure. Don't assume that your physician has already told you everything you need to know—or that you heard, understood, and remembered all of the instructions your healthcare provider gave you. Ask about pre-treatment precautions specific to your procedure. And ask well in advance; as with passports and visas, the earlier the better.

The healthier you are before your treatment, the better your chance of a positive outcome. Prior to your procedure, follow these steps:

- **Stop smoking,** as it impedes the healing process. Smoking also damages your air passages, which makes lung infections more likely. If you're planning major surgery, and particularly cosmetic surgery, your physician will insist that you stop smoking prior to the procedure.

- **Maintain a healthy weight.** Overweight patients are more prone to infection.

- **Inform your doctor of any current or recent illness.** A cold or the flu can lead to a chest infection and other complications. Let your physician know if you don't feel well.

- **If you're diabetic,** make sure that your blood sugar levels are under control.

Ask questions; voice concerns. Too often patients are timid about asking questions or raising concerns. Or smitten with a nostalgic notion of yesterday's paternal, omniscient physician, patients trust their doctors to provide them with all necessary information. Remember, times have changed, doctors are busy, and being chronically overbooked is now a routine part of their work.

Thus, especially as a medical traveler, you and your companion have a right — and an obligation! — to ask questions. If things don't feel right, voice concerns politely and firmly. Don't allow a procedure to move ahead until you feel good about the answers you receive.

If your surgeon doesn't provide much information without prompting, ask questions like these:

✦ How long is my recovery period?

✦ How much pain will I experience?

✦ What kinds of physical therapy will I require?

✦ How will I know when it's safe to take a long flight home?

✦ When I return home, how will I know when it's safe to return to my normal routine?

Your doctor should welcome such questions. If you don't understand the answers, or if you don't clearly understand your doctor's English, ask that the explanation be repeated. It's okay to be something of an annoyance. It's your health at stake, and getting this information right is essential to your well-being.

Be germ-obsessed. Whether on the streets or in a deluxe hospital suite, cleanliness is a common worry among health travelers. Food- and water-borne pathogens are a significant concern, both at home and abroad. But be reassured. Although standards of cleanliness vary from country to country (some, including Taiwan, consider Western hygienic standards inferior), infection rates in nearly all accredited hospitals abroad generally rank on par with, or a little lower than, rates in countries such as the US.

However, risk does exist in any country and any hospital, so it pays to be vigilant and follow a few simple precautions. When in the hospital, before and after treatment:

✦ Make sure that you wash your hands thoroughly, particularly after using the toilet. Remind your companion, physician, nurse, and other hospital staff to do likewise before and after attending to you. They should wear gloves. If they don't, insist that they do.

✦ Inform your nurse if the site around the needle of an IV drip is not clean and dry.

✦ Ask that hair around the site of a surgical incision be clipped, not shaven. Razors cause tiny lacerations where infections can invade.

✦ Tell your nurse if bandages or other dressings aren't clean and dry or if they are sticking to incisions. Ask that discolored, wet, or smelly dressings be changed.

✦ Ask staff members to check on tubes or catheters that feel displaced or may be malfunctioning.

✦ Do deep-breathing exercises to prevent chest infections.

✦ Ask relatives or friends who have colds or are unwell not to visit. If your companion contracts a cold or flu, postpone visits or keep them as brief as possible.

✦ Watch out for unclean clothing, floors, or instruments, and bring such breaches of hygiene to the attention of physicians or staff.

Managing post-treatment discomfort and complications. You've been out of surgery for two days, you hurt all over, your digestive system is acting up, and you're running a fever. Have you somehow contracted an antibiotic-resistant staph infection?

Coping with post-surgery discomfort is difficult enough when you're close to home. Lying for long hours in a hospital bed, far away from home and family — that's often the darkest time for a health traveler.

Knowledge is the best antidote to needless worry. As with pre-surgery preparation, ask lots of questions about post-surgery discomforts *before* heading into the operating room. Be sure to ask doctors and nurses about what kinds of discomforts to expect following your specific procedure.

If your discomfort or pain becomes acute, bleeding is persistent, or you suspect a growing infection, you may be experiencing a complication that is more serious than mere discomfort and requires immediate attention. Contact your physician without delay.

Follow doctor's orders. That advice holds for post-treatment as well as pre-treatment. Physicians the world over complain long and loud about patient noncompliance. A large number of patients — 40 percent or more according to some reports — simply will not follow the programs prescribed for them. Patients don't take their pharmaceuticals, despite clear instructions on the bottle. They don't attend physical therapy sessions, despite inarguable research that shows dramatically improved recovery rates when physical therapy is deployed. Patients don't follow instructions for bed rest, choosing instead to head back to the office prematurely or hop onto a riding lawn mower before they should. If that sounds like you, rethink your strategies — and comply! Your body, mind, and loved ones will thank you. So will your doctor.

Before Leaving the Hospital: Get All the Paperwork

Wonderful! Your treatment was a success! You've rested a little and are now more than eager to leave the hospital for the comforts of home or that luxury hotel you've booked for a much-anticipated vacation. Not so fast! Impatient to be gone, and often suffering the woozy side effects of surgery and post-operative pharmaceuticals, patients too often find themselves back at home later, missing important documents that could have more easily been obtained on site. So before you hightail it out of your hospital or clinic, be sure that you have all of your important documents.

Generally, larger hospitals provide complete medical documentation as part of the standard exit procedure. However, some smaller clinics may rely more on verbal instructions, and they are less likely to build and maintain a dossier on your case.

Regardless, be sure that you have the following in your possession before you walk out of the hospital (ideally, prior to making final payment):

✦ *Any x-rays your surgeon and staff may have taken.* Try to get all x-rays and images in digital form (.jpg or .tif files) as well as hardcopy.

✦ *Any pre- or post-operative photographs.* If your doctor doesn't take them, you might ask your companion to snap a few close-ups. While not entirely complimentary, photographs provide additional visual information for your specialists back home, as well as backup should complications arise.

> Before you hightail it out of your hospital or clinic, be sure that you have all of your important documents.

✦ *Any test results* from exams, blood work, or scans.

✦ *Post-operative instructions* (e.g., diet and physical activity precautions, bed rest, bandaging, and bathing). If your doctor doesn't furnish you with such instructions, ask for them. If you can't obtain written instructions, arrange a time to talk with your doctor and take careful notes.

✦ *Prescribed medication(s) and the written prescription(s), including instructions on dosage and duration.* If the pharmaceutical is a brand name manufactured in a country outside your own, be sure to ask your doctor what the comparable prescription is in your country. Your doctors at home may not know, and they'll feel more confident prescribing it for you if you can provide them with documentation from your overseas practitioners.

✦ *Physical therapy recommendations or prescriptions,* including full schedules and instructions.

✦ *Exit papers* that indicate your discharge with a clean bill of health.

✦ *Insurance claim forms,* if you've determined that your treatment is covered by a particular plan or for a particular hospital.

✦ *Receipts for payment,* particularly if you paid in cash.

For more on record keeping and transfer, see "Continuity of Care" in Chapter Two.

Action Item: Alert your doctor prior to treatment that you'll be requesting copies of all images, instructions, and notes. Then a medical staffer can arrange to have duplicates made for you. Alerting your doctor serves notice that you're serious about wanting documentation, and the medical staff will be more likely to assemble and duplicate all materials as treatment proceeds.

Speaking of paperwork, be sure to keep a journal near your bed, so you or your companion can easily jot notes and keep them in a central place. Keep lists of questions so you don't forget to ask them. Record all verbal instructions and important observations for future reference.

Leisure Time: Before or After Treatment?

In the words of one physician, "Minor surgery is what other people experience.

Since the recent dawn of contemporary medical travel, the media have had a field day promoting the image of sophisticated, devil-may-care patients jetsetting overseas for treatment and then heading to exotic resorts for two-week romps. Truth is, few health travelers match that description. The overwhelming majority of health travelers we interviewed had focused on researching, locating, and receiving quality healthcare at significant cost savings. Vacation and leisure time played second fiddle.

Thus, before booking a week's vacation in Taiwan, consider the following:

Intensity of treatment and length of recovery period. While promoters of health travel may imply otherwise, there's a big difference between tooth whitening and a hip replacement. Or in the words of one physician, "Minor surgery is what other people experience." When it's you, it's major, and even a simple tooth extraction or browlift involves pain, swelling, post-treatment care, pharmaceuticals, and possible complications.

If you're undergoing surgery, focus on your recuperation. If your surgeon recommends a great beachside recovery setting nearby, then all the better. In any event, even if you're planning only minor surgery, build in at least three days of recovery immediately following your treatment before heading out on a vacation.

Remember that for many surgeries — and for *all* cosmetic treatment — you are required to avoid exposure to the sun for at least two weeks.

Remember also that air travel too soon after surgery increases the risk of deep vein thrombosis (DVT), which is the formation of a clot, or thrombus, in one of the deep veins, usually in the lower leg. The immobility of long flights increases DVT risk, as does recent surgery. You can take preventive measures, including wearing compression stockings and moving about while on planes and trains. Ask your doctor about how soon after surgery you can undertake a long, sedentary trip. (For more on DVT, see Chapter Five.)

> If you don't have at least three weeks to travel, reconsider combining treatment with pleasure and focus on what's important — your health!

Your availability. Most health travel journeys take at least ten days: three or so for consultation and treatment and at least seven for recovery. Thus, if you or your companion works for a living, an extended stay may be out of the question. On the other hand, if you are retired or you have vacation days accrued, building leisure activities into the trip could be good medicine.

If you don't have at least three weeks to travel, reconsider combining treatment with pleasure and focus on what's important — your health!

Your pocketbook. The idea of saving a lot on airfare because "you're already there" is attractive. An added vacation may feel like a free bonus. But vacation expenses add up, and you're still spending real cash for every vacation day you take. Are you sure you want to spend the money you saved by getting healthcare overseas on a vacation you would never have taken otherwise? If money is tight, perhaps you're wiser to plan shorter, simpler, cheaper vacations at some other time, when you are feeling your best. Maybe the money you saved on treatment can be put to better use if saved for later. Patients who opt out of long, potentially stressful vacation trips tacked on to their health travel tend to return home in a better frame of mind—and with fewer complications.

Your personal preferences. Some health travelers we interviewed had no problem taking a week's vacation in-country before heading into the hospital for treatment. Others worried the entire time. "All I did was fret about the procedure and all the unknowns before me," said one knee-replacement patient. "I would have been better off postponing the fun part for another time."

> Patients who opt out of long, potentially stressful vacation trips tacked on to their health travel tend to return home in a better frame of mind — and with fewer complications.

Your companion. When planning your medical journey, consider your companion's interests as well as your own. One patient we interviewed found that her companion—although a great friend and ally and a huge contributor to her successful heart surgery — was not the ideal fun mate. While in Taiwan, they had different notions about what to see during their leisure time. Sharon, a history buff, wanted to visit the National Palace Museum; Marta wanted to head into the mountains to see Sun Moon Lake.

Your first priority. We found the most successful health travel vacationers were either veteran medical travelers who knew the ropes or patients who had lots of time on their hands — at least a month — to tack a vacation onto their treatment and full recovery period.

If you fall into neither of those categories, consider earmarking some of your medical savings for some delayed gratification — in the form of an unfettered, fully relaxing vacation once you've successfully recovered. Why rush it, when in truth a successful medical treatment and a fun vacation usually make for strange bedfellows? For the moment, know that most successful health travelers focus their efforts on taking care of their bodies, recovering successfully, and returning home happy and well.

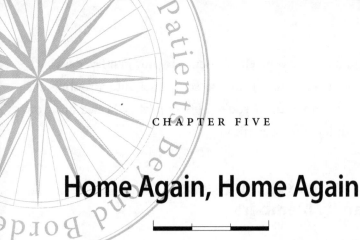

CHAPTER FIVE

Home Again, Home Again

Beating Those Home-Again Blues

It's something of a paradox: arriving home from a long trip is at once joyful — and challenging.

After all, you've just been to a new and exciting place. Perhaps the richness of culture, the cordiality of the people, or the quality of the healthcare you received surprised you. You may have delighted in learning a thing or two about Taiwan. Maybe you even picked up a bit of wanderlust on the road.

On the downside, you're probably experiencing the expected discomforts of surgery, the side effects of pharmaceuticals, and the annoyances of jet lag.

You'll likely return home exhausted, only to face backlogged bills, clogged email, endless voice-mail messages, demanding kids, and a dirty house. Take a deep breath and try to relax. It's important to pace yourself, particularly your first few days back home, allowing yourself time to settle back into a routine. It's even more important if you're not completely healed and you need additional recovery time.

Communicate Your Needs to Family Members

Yay! Dad's home! He went all the way to Taiwan for a knee replacement and came back alive to tell about it. In all the hubbub, family members also need to know that dad or mom might still need prescriptions filled, physical therapy, followup consultations with physicians, additional tests, x-rays, and lab work. You, the health traveler, may be unable to return to your full pre-treatment load of tasks and responsibilities — at least not right away. Let family members know how they can help. Accommodations — as simple as a son who does his own laundry for a while or a mother-in-law who brings over a casserole — can make a world of difference.

Action Item: **Within a day or two after returning from your trip, review your exit documentation carefully with your family and loved ones, and clearly communicate the help you need to complete a successful recovery. If possible, form a plan of who will do what, whether it's tracking down a prescription, giving you a lift to the local occupational therapy center, or simply loading the dishwasher after dinner.**

Touch Base with Your Local Doctor

If you followed our advice in previous chapters, you informed your local doctor or specialist about your health trip *prior* to departure. When you sent your medical records abroad, you established the basis for a continuing communication between your local healthcare provider and your overseas physician (see "Continuity of Care" in Chapter Two).

Shortly after your return, pay a brief visit (or send an email) to your healthcare provider's office and let everyone there know that you're back. Chances are you'll have specific needs, based on your overseas physician's instructions or recommendations. You might need an antibiotic prescription refilled or six weeks of physical therapy approved. Thus, it's best to touch base as soon as you reasonably can, both as a courtesy and for practical reasons.

Most physicians will be understanding and cooperative, particularly if you've brought home complete, accurate paperwork. If for some reason you find your physician uncooperative or uncommunicative, then consider seeking another healthcare provider sooner rather than later. So make that call to your hometown doc soon after returning home.

Anticipate Longer Recovery Periods

Whether treated at home or abroad, most patients can expect recovery periods of three months — sometimes even more — for large, invasive surgeries. For less stringent procedures, recovery periods range from a few days to several weeks. Regardless of the intensity of your treatment, don't be surprised if you find that you need what seems like a long time to feel fully yourself again, particularly after a long trip.

It's easy, for example, to underestimate the effects of jet lag. In fact, seasoned travelers know that, for every one hour of time zone difference, travelers should allow one day to fully recover from jet lag. For a trip to Asia, that's nearly two weeks! Typical jet lag discomforts include feelings of disorientation, fatigue, and general tiredness, inability to sleep, loss of concentration, loss of drive, headaches, upset stomach, and a general feeling of unwellness.

> Seasoned travelers know that, for every one hour of time zone difference, travelers should allow one day to fully recover from jet lag.

Add symptoms of jet lag to the list of unavoidable post-treatment discomforts, and your body's inner voices will be pleading with you to take things easy, at least during the first week after your return.

At home, some patients feel timid about asking for help, particularly if they managed to work a vacation or extended recovery period into the trip. Yet the fact remains that the healing body needs a great deal of rest and attention. Don't be afraid to voice a gentle reminder that you're still recuperating.

Hold On to Your Paperwork

Remember all that paperwork and assorted gobbledygook the hospital gave you prior to your departure? Forms, instructions, prescriptions, notes, and recommendations *ad nauseum* — keep it all! Take it with you when you visit your local doctor, who's likely to find those documents more informative and reliable than your personal account of the trip. If your physician wants to keep any of the documents, ask for a copy for your files.

Action Item: **Comply with your doctors' instructions before, during, and after any procedure. Every single one of them.**

Stay with the Program

We've said it elsewhere in the book: pre- and post-procedure, it's all about compliance, compliance, compliance.

If you've just had dental surgery, you might be instructed to use a special antiseptic rinse twice a day. Do so. Or after an orthopedic procedure, patients are usually required to undergo a rigorous physical therapy program. Do that, too. Nearly all procedures come with a regimen of antibiotics and other prescriptions, sometimes lasting weeks. That means you!

Granted, it's no fun to take those big horse capsules or drag yourself to that physical therapy appointment when you really need to clear those 400 emails sitting in your inbox. But consider the alternative: after all that work and investment and travel, do you really want to develop complications that could cost you extra time and money — if not your life?

Fully inform your family members and close friends about your post-treatment procedures and regimens. Loved ones should encourage you to do everything you can to get better, and they should help you follow your program in every way possible. Pepper your calendar and to-do list with reminders — of your medications, appointments, therapy sessions, and other health-promoting activities.

Get Help or Farm Out the Work

If you've come this far in your health travel experience, chances are you're one of those people who "do it all." You're good at planning and problem-solving, juggling many balls at once, keeping myriad tasks and projects in the air, and walking the tightrope of a complex contemporary life. That's why an otherwise challenging, difficult journey turned out so well. You managed it!

Now that you're home, cut yourself some slack. Don't try to return immediately to your pre-treatment pace. If housecleaning was one of your daily chores, use some of your treatment savings to hire a temporary maid service. If you need to repair a lawn mower so you can cut the grass, send it into the shop. You get the idea. For the first month or so after your trip, demand less of yourself and work back gradually into your normal routine.

> For the first month or so after your trip, demand less of yourself and work back gradually into your normal routine.

Stay Mentally and Socially Active

During a long recovery period, it's easy to become bored, isolated, and listless, falling into a rut of watching endless TV or surfing the Internet for hours on end. If your recovery doesn't allow you to be as physically active as you'd like or to return to work immediately, try to stay as emotionally fit as possible. Get a friend to bring you a stack of your favorite reading materials from the local library. Invite friends and family members to watch a good movie with you. Take up chess again, or Dungeons and Dragons, or whatever activity keeps you stimulated. Studies show that patients who stay mentally and socially active post-treatment recover better and faster than those who become couch potatoes.

> Studies show that patients who stay mentally and socially active post-treatment recover better and faster than those who become couch potatoes.

If Complications Develop . . .

If your doctors in Taiwan played your treatment by the rules, they probably insisted that you remain in-country for at least a few days following your procedure. The main reason was to observe your progress and monitor your condition for any signs of complications, which are more serious than the usual discomforts experienced post-surgery. Most complications arise within a week after surgery. While 95 percent of all surgical patients experience no post-treatment complications, every patient should be able to recognize the warning signs and promptly seek medical help.

Post-Treatment: Normal Discomfort or Something More Complicated?

Prior to your surgery, your doctor should thoroughly explain the procedure and tell you about any discomforts you can expect after being wheeled out of the operating unit. Discomforts differ from complications. Discomforts are predictable and unthreatening. Complications, while rarely life-threatening, are more serious and may require prompt medical attention.

These are some common discomforts you can expect following your surgery:

+ Minor local pain and general achiness

+ Swelling (after dentistry)

+ Puffiness (after cosmetic surgery)

+ Bruising, swelling, or minor bleeding around an incision

+ Headaches (side effect of anesthesia)

+ Urinary retention, or difficulty urinating (side effect of anesthesia and catheters)

+ Nausea and vomiting, headache, dry mouth, temporary loss of memory, lingering tiredness (all common side effects of anesthesia)

+ Hunger and under-nutrition

Most surgically induced discomforts recede or disappear altogether during the first few days after treatment, as the body and spirit return to normal. Be sure to report discomforts that persist or become more pronounced, as they might be early warning signs of more serious complications.

Complications vary according to each type of surgery, and you should be aware of the more common ones. Complications are scary, and many doctors would rather not go into morbid detail about them unless pressed. Complications are rare; most arise in less than 5 percent of total cases — and generally among patients who are aged or infirm in the first place. So while it's wise to be informed and vigilant, there's no need to worry yourself sick anticipating the worst.

Common symptoms of complications include

✦ Infection, increased pain, or swelling around an incision

✦ Abnormal bleeding around an incision

✦ Sudden or unexplained high fever

✦ Extreme chest pain or shortness of breath

✦ Extreme headache

✦ Extreme difficulty urinating

If you experience any of the symptoms listed above, call your hometown physician immediately.

Caution: Blood Clots in the Veins

Air travel after surgery may put you at risk of deep vein thrombosis (DVT), a term that describes the formation of a clot, or thrombus, in one of the deep veins, usually in the lower leg. The immobility of long flights increases the risk, as does recent surgery. The symptoms of DVT may include pain and redness of the skin over a vein or swelling and tenderness in the ankle, foot, or thigh. More serious symptoms include chest pain and shortness of breath.

You can take preventive measures to reduce your risk of DVT. Wear compression stockings and move about frequently while on planes and trains. Ask your doctor about how soon after surgery you can undertake a long, sedentary trip.

Other Ways to Reduce DVT Risk

Before you travel:

✦ Stop smoking.

✦ Lose weight if you need to.

✦ Get enough exercise to be at least minimally fit before your surgery and your travel.

✦ Discuss stopping birth control pills and hormone replacement therapy with your doctor.

✦ Travel on an airline that provides sufficient leg room.

✦ Wear loose clothing.

✦ Reserve an aisle seat on the airplane so you can get up and move around easily.

✦ Ask your surgeon about using a pneumatic compression device during and after surgery.

✦ Before your return flight home, ask your surgeon if you need an anticoagulant.

✦ Walk briskly for at least half an hour before takeoff.

On the plane:

✦ Don't stow your carry-on luggage under your seat if it restricts your movement.

✦ Flex your calves and rotate your ankles every 20–30 minutes.

✦ Walk up and down the aisle every two hours or less.

✦ Sleep only for short periods.

✦ Do not take sleeping pills.

✦ Drink lots of water to avoid dehydration.

✦ Avoid alcohol, caffeine, and diet soda.

✦ Wear elastic flight socks or support stockings.

✦ Don't let your stockings or clothing roll up or constrict your legs.

✦ Take deep breaths frequently throughout your flight.

The Straight Dope on Pharmaceuticals

rue or false: When traveling, it's okay to bring small amounts of prescription drugs back into your home country.

True or false: It's legal to order prescriptions from reputable online pharmacies outside your country.

Believe it or not—for many Western countries—the answer is false on both counts, though with some favorable caveats!

Many international travelers like to purchase their favorite prescriptions less expensively while abroad. While it's *technically* illegal in the US and some other countries, consumer activists have turned the issue into a political hot potato. Consequently, at this writing, customs inspectors are often reluctant to bust granny with her two vials of benazepril, and in most instances they turn a blind eye to folks entering the country with prescription drugs purchased abroad. Thus, it's become a gray area, with customs inspectors empowered to use "general discretion" when prescription drugs are found. Most often, the offending pharmaceuticals are simply confiscated, and the traveler must decide whether it's worth struggling with all the red tape required to petition for their return.

The overwhelming number of tourists carrying pharmaceuticals purchased abroad enter the country with no trouble, usually unnoticed. The best advice is to use common sense. You're far less likely to be hassled for carrying a single prescription's worth of amoxicillin than if your suitcase is seen bursting with enough tramadol to supply the streets of Los Angeles for a year. And as always, if you're carrying drugs that are illegal—prescription or otherwise—you may be subject to arrest, as well as seizure of the prohibited items.

Similarly, it's *technically* illegal in the US and some other countries to purchase any pharmaceutical of any kind from any mail-order pharmacy outside the country. Again, highly vocal activists have prevailed politically in the US and elsewhere, and only a small fraction of prescription drugs purchased from foreign countries are seized. In those cases, the pharmacies often double-ship the order, so the buyer usually doesn't even know the purchase was interrupted.

Until the laws change, you're advised to use good judgment on this issue as well. Purchase only from reputable pharmacies, using legitimate prescriptions from your physician. And anticipate the outside chance you'll be among the few every year who are inconvenienced by seizures of prescription drugs.

It's perfectly legal to purchase prescription medications online from authorized mail-order pharmacies inside your home country.

For specifics about importing controlled substances into the US, call 1 202 307.2414. US citizens can obtain additional information about traveling with medication from any FDA office, or they can write to the US Food and Drug Administration, Division of Import Operations and Policy, Room 12-8 (HFC-170), 5600 Fishers Lane, Rockville, MD 20857. For further information on prescription drug rules and regulations, US citizens can contact the FDA's Center for Drugs, 1 888 INFO.FDA (toll-free) or www.fda.gov/cder. Citizens of other countries are encouraged to contact the appropriate government office for full rules and regulations.

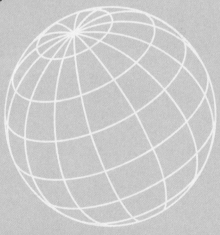

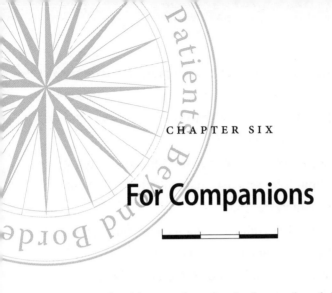

For Companions

"Hold a true friend in both your hands."
— Nigerian proverb

Joining a friend, family member, or other loved one on a medical journey is truly a gift, but the rewards are many. Some companions simply appreciate the opportunity to travel. Others enjoy the chance to spend one-on-one time with a person who is important to them, perhaps to deepen a relationship. With most companions, there's an element of being "in this together" — working through a unique experience and its inevitable surprises, then heading home with great stories to tell!

First Things First: Are You Up for the Job?

Before you overthink that question, here's some succinct advice: go with your first instincts.

If you've already agreed to be a companion health traveler and you've not been bribed, railroaded, or otherwise coerced into the job, then chances are your first impressions were correct. While the journey won't always be a cakewalk, most memorable worthwhile experiences are less than easy, and they're the stuff of profound and lasting memories.

If you've been asked to be a companion and are having strong reservations about it for any reason, then either talk it out with your friend or politely decline.

If you're on the fence about being a companion, you might want to flip through Chapter Two, "Planning Your Health Travel Journey," where you'll find important criteria for a successful companion-patient relationship. In brief, if you're reliable, orga- nized, and like to have some fun, chances are good you and your partner will be enriched for the experience, despite — and often because of — the rough patches you'll inevitably encounter.

Know there are no magic formulas, although a good dose of common sense mixed with empathy and attentiveness is the main initial requirement. Each patient is different, as is each relationship between patient and companion. Use the sections below to get an idea of the broad requirements and the journey's milestones, and the rest will follow.

Before the Trip

The devil of any medical trip is in the details. The more of them you and your partner nail down before boarding the plane, the more successful the trip and treatment will be. Patients are often distracted prior to the trip, not only by the usual family and pro- fessional concerns, but also by perfectly understandable worries about their upcoming treatment and travel. A good companion can help keep heads together, maintain calm in the household, and expedite trip planning greatly.

Use the checklist below to make sure that either you or your partner has addressed each important preparation:

+ **Passports and visas.** At least a month prior to your departure, check to see that you and your partner either have them or that they're on order. Just before your departure, make sure both of you carry them on your person — don't leave them on the dining room table. You won't need a visa for a trip to Taiwan if you are a citizen of Australia, Austria, Belgium, Canada, Costa Rica, New Zealand, Norway, Portugal, Singapore, the UK, or the US. Medical travelers can arrange for six-month visas if needed.

> The devil of any medical trip is in the details. The more of them you and your partner nail down before boarding the plane, the more successful the trip and treatment will be.

+ **Medical documentation.** Make sure the health traveler has packed all written diagnoses, treatment recommendations, cost estimates, x-rays, lab reports, blood test results, and any other information related to the treatment — even if copies of this information have already been sent overseas. Your partner's in-country physician and staff may need them, and taking them will save you time and money.

+ **Kids, cats, and newspaper delivery.** Work with your partner to make sure all the family living arrangements are in order, and ask frequently how you can help. Examples of services you might provide include finding a pet sitter, making sure bills are paid in advance, and suspending newspaper delivery.

✦ **Confirm and reconfirm appointments and reservations.** A couple of days prior to departure, call or email the physician and treatment center to reconfirm all appointments and scheduled treatments. Do the same for your flight reservations, lodging, and any local transportation you've booked.

✦ **Read up on your destination.** If you can spare the time, become acquainted with Taiwan or any other destination you choose. Check your local library for travel guides, skim them for content, make notes, and then buy the one you and your partner like best. Or do an Internet search for the city and country where you'll be staying, print what interests you, and toss the print-out into your travel bag.

> If you learn some facts about the culture and history, the local people will invariably appreciate your interest.

Although you need not be fluent in the language, at least one of you should know a little something about the local customs, protocol, transportation, restaurants, and historic sites. If you learn some facts about the culture and history, the local people will invariably appreciate your interest. That goes double if you manage to learn even a few words of the language.

✦ **Prescriptions and other essentials.** While you can purchase just about anything abroad that you might have forgotten to pack, some things are more easily replaced than others, especially on a medical trip. Don't worry about a comb or shampoo, but make sure you and your partner have packed important medications and prescriptions, an extra set of eyeglasses if you wear them, plus special creams, medicinal soaps, hard-to-find ointments, and the like. Thoroughly check the medicine cabinet and bathroom counter to make sure you've packed all the creature comforts and necessities that might be difficult to purchase abroad. In these days of tight airport security, it's best to pack liquids and gels in checked luggage, but keep prescription medicines (in their original containers) in your carry-on bag.

> Spell out expectations. For example, who's paying for the airfare? Lodging and meals? Sightseeing and tours?

✦ *Finances.* Sometimes even the best of friends can encounter misunderstandings about who is to pay for what. Avoid damaging your relationship by addressing financial questions early. Spell out expectations. For example, who's paying for the airfare? Lodging and meals? Sightseeing and tours?

Generally, with the more expensive surgeries (e.g., cardiovascular and orthopedic), the cost of a companion is factored into the overall savings of the procedure. However, a tooth cleaning and whitening that's more vacation than medical journey might entail a different set of financial parameters and expectations. In any event, get it straight before the trip, and you'll both breathe easier.

While You're There

Once you've landed, a zillion challenges large and small will confront you, and they can be disconcerting, especially if you're not accustomed to traveling. That is where travel partners are either at their best or at their worst with each other. Keep your cool. Take a deep breath. Seasoned travelers know to "go with the flow" and have faith that all will turn out well. It usually does.

At the airport. Even if you are a seasoned international traveler, touchdown at your in-country destination is likely to be the most challenging part of your trip. You've just arrived in a strange land full of oddly dressed people who are moving about with a lot more confidence than you are. You're exhausted and grimy from the trip; the only things on your mind are a shower and a bed. But you have things you must do first. Keep your wits, snag some local currency from the airport money exchange, suffer your way through immigration and customs, gather *all* your luggage, find your transportation, and make a beeline for your hotel or treatment center. After that, the worst is behind you.

Hospital check-in. Hospitals and clinics can be chaotic, bewildering places until you learn your way around. Two sets of eyes — and vocal cords — are better than one. Most often you'll be pleasantly surprised by the level of attention and care given to international health travelers. In the unlikely event that you're not getting the service you need, gently, but firmly, find the right personnel and make sure you're noticed and served. If not, contact your physician or travel broker directly.

Pre-treatment. Once checked in at the hospital or hotel, companions can turn their attention to providing emotional support, easing pre-treatment jitters, and doing little things to help the health traveler settle comfortably into unfamiliar surroundings and circumstances. Order flowers for the room? Draw a relaxing bath?

Probably more than any other time spent in-country, the period between the hospital check-in and the procedure itself requires the greatest vigilance and the largest number of quick decisions. During this brief time, both you and the patient will be meeting with doctors and staff, becoming acquainted with the facilities, and deriving a mutual understanding about what to expect in the coming days and weeks.

During this period, it's not uncommon for health travelers to experience doubts and second thoughts. It's natural to wonder if a huge life mistake has been made, particularly when far from the comforts of home and family.

> Generally, if the surroundings are clean, the staff attentive, and the physicians and surgeons communicative, you and your partner have little to worry about.

Generally, if the surroundings are clean, the staff attentive, and the physicians and surgeons communicative, you and your partner have little to worry about. You'll find that your misgivings are like passing storms — turbulent and upsetting, and then followed by calm and bright light. However, if you and your partner have persistent concerns, particularly about hospital hygiene, staff competence, or treatment outcomes, voice them immediately. Or if you feel that important facts have been misrepresented (such as physician's credentials, hospital accreditation, or surgery success rates), arrange additional consultations until you've resolved the problem. No patient should venture into treatment until reasonable trust has been established with the physician and other healthcare providers.

Post-treatment. Even after the least invasive procedures, patients experience discomfort, even pain. Your partner will also probably experience disorientation from medications, particularly if painkillers are involved. This is the time to be extremely sympathetic and attentive. During the first few days after treatment, patients often encounter discouragement, irritability, and sometimes-unnerving mood swings. This is normal for any treatment and more so when recuperating far from the comforts of home.

This phase passes. The trauma and discomfort of the treatment become more familiar and manageable, the pain recedes, and you both become more comfortable in your surroundings. During those initial days post-treatment, a little positive thinking goes a long way.

Here's how you can help in the days immediately following treatment:

Have big ears. Listen carefully to advice and directives given by physicians and staff, and then follow them. Your partner may be unable to retain it all. You might need to head out and fill a prescription or two. Or maybe the respiratory therapist didn't show up, and you need to find out why. Or the doctor gave orders for two days of ice-pack treatment, but the ice hasn't materialized. Medical directives in a hospital or clinic are often verbal. The more of them you remember and act on, the better the patient's prognosis.

Help stay in touch with friends and family. Just when loved ones at home are most concerned about the outcome, your partner may not yet feel up to talking on the phone or sitting at a computer and tapping out a reassuring email. When you have a good grasp on how things are going, ask your partner if it's all right for you to get in touch with family and friends. Often just a call or two will reassure the folks back home, who will appreciate hearing news from afar.

> During the first few days after treatment, patients often encounter discouragement, irritability, and sometimes-unnerving mood swings. This is normal for any treatment and more so when recuperating far from the comforts of home.

Get away. As helpful and needed as you are, you're not super-human. You, too, require time for yourself—so take it! Find an afternoon or a day to get away from the hospital or hotel. With a little research, you'll quickly find a rich array of nearby, easily accessible excursions. If you like city life and shopping, Taipei 101 may be just what you are looking for. Located in the fashionable Xinyi district, this renowned commercial hotspot overflows with high-end brands, such as Chanel, Gucci, and Coach. If getting out to the countryside is more to your liking, plan a trip to Taroko Gorge with its sharply rising cliffs, verdant riverbed, and mountain hiking trails. These little sojourns will help rejuvenate you, and you'll return home with some colorful memories of your visit.

Back Home

Be in contact often. If you're a spouse or close family member who's gone along as a health traveler's companion, then you may resume living under the same roof when you return home and maintaining contact isn't a problem. But friends who served as travel companions may need to make more effort. As life at home quickly gives way to daily routine, it's comforting for the patient to hear the travel companion's voice or see that friendly, reassuring face occasionally. So check in from time to time, ask if there's anything you can do, and simply be a friend. Recovery is often a lonely period for a patient, who, despite all other indications, isn't quite ready yet to rejoin the real world.

> As helpful and needed as you are, you're not superhuman. You, too, require time for yourself — so take it!

Help promote compliance. Good post-treatment compliance is the best way to prevent complications and ensure a fast, full recovery. As one who lived and breathed the patient's experience and heard the doctor's orders first-hand, you're best equipped to prod your partner into maximal compliance with every part of the post-treatment program.

Encourage family members and friends to participate. Even if you live under the same roof with the patient, you can't do it all. So, encourage those closest to your partner to participate. Spread out the work by assigning specific tasks, such as bathing, bandage changing, or transport to post-treatment consultations and physical therapy appointments. Sometimes friends and family want to be helpful but don't know what they can do. Your insider's understanding of the patient's needs can work wonders during the important first weeks after the trip.

Help your partner stay physically, mentally, and socially active. After treatment, some patients lapse into relative isolation and inactivity, particularly if they weren't athletic or social in the first place. Get your partner up and out for a walk around the block, offer gentle reminders about church or school events, and do everything you can to keep the recovering health traveler functional and alert.

Action Item: **Help your partner stay mentally and physically active during the recovery period.**

A Note to Patients about Your Companion

A person who joins you on a medical trip is the best friend you have in the world. Respect the gift. Both of you will be in a new land, trying to process a bewildering range of new experiences while facing serious concerns about your health and your immediate future. During those challenging moments that confront every health traveler, take it easy on one another and keep the faith that all will turn out well.

When you have specific wants or needs, express them to your companion as clearly as you can. Take the time to verbalize your appreciation for your companion's presence. He or she made a big effort to join you — gave a large and true gift of love. Be as gentle and patient as possible with one another, and the deepened kinship fashioned from your travel experience will be its own reward.

Dos and Don'ts
for the Smart Health Traveler

Much of the advice in this chapter is covered in greater detail elsewhere in this book. Consider this a capsule summary of essential information, sprinkled with practical advice that will help reduce the number of inevitable "gotchas" that health travelers encounter. You may want your travel companion and family members to read this chapter, along with the Introduction to Part One, so they better understand medical travel. They can use this information as a gateway to the more in-depth sections of this book.

✔ *Do* Plan Ahead

Particularly if you'll be traveling at peak tourist season, the further in advance you plan, the more likely you are to get the best doctors, the lowest airfares, and the best availability and rates on lodging. Remember, you'll be competing for treatment with other health travelers. You'll also be competing with tourists for hotels and transportation. If possible, begin planning at least three months prior to your expected departure date. If you're concerned about having to change plans, *do* be sure to confirm cancellation policies with airlines, hotels, and travel agents. For more information, see Chapter Two, "Planning Your Health Travel Journey."

✔ *Do* Be Sure about Your Diagnosis and Treatment Preference

The more you know about the treatment you're seeking, the easier your search for a physician will be. For example, if you're seeking dental work, you should know specifically whether you want implants or bridgework. If the former, then you'll be narrowing your search to accredited implantologists. *Do* work closely with your hometown doctor or medical specialist, and make sure you obtain exact recommendations — in writing, if possible. If you are unsure of your needs or not confident of your doctor's diagnosis, seek a second opinion. Then, when you know your specific course of action, learn as much as you can about your procedure using textbooks, medical references, and reliable sites on the Internet. For more information on recommended health research sites, see Part Four, "Resources and References," in the back of the book.

✔ *Do* Research Your In-Country Doctor Thoroughly

This is the most important step of all. By following a few basic guidelines, you'll see the process is not daunting. When you've narrowed your search to two or three physicians, invest time and money in personal telephone interviews or teleconferences, either directly with the doctors or through the hospital's international patients coordinator. *Don't* be afraid to ask questions — lots of them — until you arrive at a comfort level with a competent physician. For more information, see Chapter Two.

✘ *Don't* Rely Completely on the Internet for Your Research

While the online world has matured over the last few years, searching for information isn't yet on automatic pilot. Deeper digging — and more effort on your part — are usually required. While it's okay to use the Web for your initial research, *don't* assume that Web sites offer complete and accurate information. Cross-check your online findings with referrals, articles in leading newspapers and magazines, and word-of-mouth reports. You'll begin to find the same names of clinics and physicians popping up. Narrow your search from there.

✔ *Do* Get It in Writing

Cost estimates, appointments, recommendations, opinions, second opinions, air and hotel accommodations — get as much as you can in writing, and *do* be sure to take all documentation with you on the plane. Email is fine, as long as you've retained a printed record of your key transactions. If you prefer to use the telephone, confirm your conversation(s) with a followup email: "As we discussed, it's my understanding that the cost for my treatment, including _____ and _____ will be US$20,000. Is that correct? Could you please confirm that in a letter or email?" The more you get in writing, the less the chance of a misunderstanding, particularly when confronting language and cultural barriers.

✔ *Do* Insist on English

As much as many of us would like to have a better command of another language, the time to brush up on your Mandarin Chinese is most definitely *not* when negotiating a heart bypass operation in Taipei!

As you begin your research into a medical trip, consider the language barrier as an early warning sign in your screening process. If a clinic, physician, or hospital that claims to serve international patients doesn't have a good grasp of English, then politely apologize for your lack of language skills and move on. Establishing a comfortable, reliable rapport with your key contacts is paramount to your success as a health traveler.

✘ *Don't* Schedule Your Trip Too Tightly

Most veteran health travelers admit that one of their biggest surprises was the efficiency of medical service they received while abroad. Staff-to-patient ratios in Taiwan are generally lower than in many Western hospitals, and the level of personal commitment is often higher. Yet, it's best not to plan your trip with military precision. A missed consultation or an extra two days of recovery overseas can mean rescheduling that nonrefundable airfare, with penalties. More important, scheduling a little leeway lets everyone breathe more easily and gives you the flexibility of adapting seamlessly when things don't go precisely as planned.

A good rule of thumb is to add one more day for every five days you've already scheduled for consultation, treatment, and recovery. If you're planning a facelift and tummy tuck, consultation and surgery might require three days, with a recommended recovery of ten days (totaling 13 days). Thus, you should add two or three more days to your travel schedule to allow for weather delays, missed appointments, additional tests, and other unexpected events.

✗ *Don't* Forget to Alert Your Bank and Credit Card Company

The consumer fraud units of banks and credit card institutions have recently deployed hair-trigger monitoring for unusual spending activity. Thus, overseas travelers — just when they need their credit cards and ATM cards the most — often find their accounts canceled immediately after using them in-country. Then the fun begins, as you try to connect with your bank's voice-activated customer service line, using your new overseas cell phone!

The easy fix is to contact your bank and credit card company (or companies) *prior to your trip.* Inform them of your travel dates, and tell them where you will be. If you plan to use your credit card for large amounts, alert the company in advance. Also, if you plan to use your credit card to pay for expensive treatments, this might be a good time to reconfirm your credit limits.

✔ *Do* Learn a Little about Taiwan

Once you've settled on Taiwan as your health travel destination, spend a little time getting to know something about the country. You'll find a little knowledge goes a long way: the locals will differentiate you from less caring travelers and express sincere appreciation for your interest. *Do* buy or borrow a couple of travel guides, learn a little history, and practice a few basic phrases (such as hello, goodbye, please, thank you, excuse me). When in Taiwan, pick up an English-language newspaper, which will get you up to speed on current events, happenings around town, and local gossip.

✔ *Do* Inform Your Local Doctors Before You Leave

Telling your doctor you're planning to travel overseas for treatment is a little like calling your auto mechanic to say you're taking your business to a competitor down the road. However, although you may never again see your former car mechanic, you *do* want to preserve a good working relationship with your family physician and local specialists.

Although they may not particularly like your decision, most doctors will respect your desire to travel overseas for medical care. Even if they privately question your judgment, they will appreciate learning about your plans *prior to* your trip. This pre-trip notification will pay off for you, too. When you return, you won't have to make an awkward call just when you most need a prescription refilled. If your physician attempts to dissuade you, *do* be attentive and polite, but stay firm in your resolve if you've done your homework and made your choice. For more on this topic, see "Continuity of Care" in Chapter Two.

✗ *Don't* Scrimp on Lodging

Unless your finances absolutely demand it, avoid hotels and other accommodations in the "budget" category. Taiwan's hotels are divided into three classes: international tourist class, tourist class, and ordinary. Legally licensed hotels post their certifications, and most health travelers should make sure that their accommodations have earned the highest rating. Even for some of Taiwan's best hotels, prices are moderate by Western standards.

✗ *Don't* Stay Too Far from Your Treatment Center

When booking hotel accommodations for you and your companion, make sure the hospital or doctor's office is nearby. This is doubly true in large cities, such as Taipei. While in-town trans-portation costs are usually low, traffic and noise levels can be horrendous, and a long, stop-and-start cross-town trip can be as stressful as a 24-hour flight. Check with your doctor, hospital, or treatment center for appropriately located lodging (see recom-mendations in Part Three).

✔ *Do* Befriend Staff

Nurses, nurse's aides, paramedics, receptionists, clerks, and even maintenance people — consider each of them a vital member of your health team! Often overlooked and always overworked, these professionals are omnipresent in the day-to-day operation of a hospital or clinic, and they wield a good deal of quiet power. You and your companion might find you need one of these folks most in the wee hours when no one else is around. Invariably, it will be the second-floor lobby clerk who knows how to get in touch with your doctor or the nightshift nurse's assistant who fetches a clean bedsheet.

You and your companion should take the time to chat with medical staff members, learn their names, inquire about their families, and proffer any small gifts you might have brought. Above all, treat staff with deference and respect. When you're ready to leave the hospital, a heartfelt thank-you note and a mod-est cash tip makes a great farewell.

✗ *Don't* Return Home Too Soon

After a long flight to a foreign land, multiple consultations with physicians and staff, and a painful and disorienting medical procedure, most folks feel ready to jump on the first flight home. That's understandable but not advisable. Your body needs time to recuperate, and your physician needs to track your recovery progress. As you plan your trip, ask your physician how much recovery time is advised for your particular treatment. Then add a few extra days, just to be on the safe side.

✗ *Don't* Be Too Adventurous with Local Cuisine

Deep-fried frogs in garlic! Angelica duck! Oyster omelet! Yes, it's true that Taiwan has robust, tasty cuisine, with a variety of local culinary fare to tempt nearly any palate. But one sure way to get your treatment off to a bad start is to enter your clinic with a rising case of traveler's diarrhea or even a mild dose of stomach upset due to local water or food intolerance.

So, when hunger calls, go easy with your food choices. Prior to treatment, avoid rich, spicy foods, exotic drinks (no ice!), and raw fruits and vegetables. If you're staying in the hospital as an inpatient, don't be afraid to ask the dietician for a menu that's easy on your digestion. Use only bottled water, even when brushing your teeth, and make sure the seal is intact. If you are healthy and feeling adventurous after your treatment, you might want to sample some of the tempting local fare, but avoid street vendors. Trust well-established, reputable restaurants for the highest quality and safest food.

Finally, find out about food interactions for any pharmaceuticals you're taking before or after your procedure. Some drugs don't work—or become downright risky—if certain foods are consumed. In short, play it safe on your medical trip; your digestive tract will thank you.

✔ *Do* Set Aside Some of Your Medical Travel Savings for a Vacation

You and your companion deserve it! If you're not able to take leisure time during your trip abroad, then set aside the extra dollars for some time off after you return home, even if only for a weekend getaway. You've demonstrated great courage and perseverance in making a difficult trip abroad, and you've earned some downtime with your cost savings.

✘ *Don't* Ever Settle for Second Best in Treatment Options

While you can cut corners on airfare, lodging, and transportation, always, always insist upon the very best healthcare your money can buy. Go the extra mile to find that best physician or surgeon. Although everyone likes a bargain, the best treatment doesn't always come from the lowest bidder. Focus on quality, not just price.

✔ *Do* Get All Your Paperwork Before Leaving the Country

Understandably, after you've undergone a treatment — whether a simple root canal or a hip replacement — you're eager to get home, go on vacation, or just get your life back. Too often and in too much of a hurry to leave, patients exit their treatment center lacking instructions, prescriptions, and other essential paperwork. Get copies of everything. For more information, see Chapter Four, "While You're There."

✔ *Do* Trust Your Intuition

Your courage and good judgment have brought you this far. Continue to rely on your sixth sense throughout your trip. If, for example, you feel uncomfortable with your in-country consultation, switch doctors. If you get a queasy feeling about extra or uncharted costs, don't be afraid to question them. Thousands of health travelers have beaten a successful path abroad, using good information and common sense. If you've come this far, chances are good you'll join their ranks.

Safe travels!

PART TWO

Taiwan's Most-Traveled
Health Destinations

Why Travel to Taiwan for Healthcare?

Tourists to Taiwan take home memories to last a lifetime: the night lights of Kaohsiung seen from a boat on the Love River; the ascent from sea level to high mountains on the Alishan Forest Railway; and the bright sunshine, blue waters, and clean sandy beaches of Kenting. Medical travelers to Taiwan return home with different kinds of memories, perhaps less picturesque but equally important: competent doctors, clean and modern hospitals, skilled nurses, friendly staff, and a successful medical procedure followed by a successful recovery.

The reasons why Western health travelers journey to Taiwan are as diverse as the travelers themselves, but the central incentive for all is the excellence of the nation's healthcare. That excellence grows from six main strengths: high quality, modern technology, patient-oriented services, a professional team approach, a comprehensive scope of medical services — and of course, affordability.

High Quality

The high quality of medical care at most hospitals in Taiwan is ensured by the Department of Health through the Taiwan Joint Commission on Hospital Accreditation (TJCHA), which visits and evaluates each facility every three years.

Taiwan's many international recognitions in this area include the following:

✦ 1996: Taiwan initiated the International Quality Indicator Project; now 76 hospitals in Taiwan participate.

✦ 2000: A leading research and advisory firm, the Economist Intelligence Unit, ranked Taiwan's healthcare as second best in the world, behind only Sweden.

✦ 2006: TJCHA's accreditation system was the eighth in the world to be accredited by the International Society for Quality in Health Care (ISQua) International Accreditation Program.

✦ 2006: Min-Sheng General Hospital and Wan Fang Medical Center were the first two hospitals in Taiwan to be awarded Joint Commission International (JCI) accreditation; eight additional hospitals are currently preparing to apply or applying for JCI accreditation.

✦ 2006: The *American Journal of Transplantation* reported that the five-year survival rate for recipients of living-donor liver transplants in Taiwan's hospitals averaged 91.2 percent, the highest in the world.

✦ Many hospitals in Taiwan participate in the World Health Organization (WHO) Health-Promoting Hospital Certification program.

✦ Laboratories in Taiwan's hospitals go through the College of American Pathologists Laboratory Accreditation Program (CAP-LAP).

✦ The citation frequency of Taiwan's published articles in clinical medicine is currently ranked twenty-first among the world's 194 nations.

Modern Technology

Taiwan's hospitals have state-of-the-art equipment that is at least equivalent, and sometimes superior, to the equipment in US hospitals. Effective use of technology reduces patients' waiting time and increases their treatment options. According to a 2007 report by the Taiwan Task Force on Medical Travel (TTFMT), Taiwan has 33 positron emission tomography (PET), 115 magnetic resonance imaging (MRI), and 321 computed tomography (CT) scanners. Also in regular use are volume-computed tomography (VCT), argon-helium cryoablation, CyberKnife, an Internet-based picture archiving and communication system (IPACS), WiMAX technology (mobile devices to monitor health indicators), and medical applications of radiofrequency identification.

Patient-Oriented Services

Providing customer-oriented, compassionate service is an important mission throughout Taiwan's healthcare system. All healthcare professionals in Taiwan believe that life is priceless, so they exert themselves to provide patient-centered care. Many hospitals, for example, offer independent health examination buildings, door-to-door service, a personal healthcare team, online message response, in-person physician consultations, English-speaking medical staff, individual translation services, international patient service centers, and five-star wards.

Professional Team Approach

In Taiwan, all healthcare personnel are fully educated and trained. Their education includes humanitarian medicine, and their services focus on the welfare and security of their patients. Doctors in Taiwan go through a varied and strict program of medical education; generally, medical students train for more than ten years to become attending physicians. Taiwan's medical groups offer the safest and most effective treatment for each individual. Friendly, caring, and competent service is central to the professional healthcare team's approach. For international patients, bilingual staff members ensure frequent and accurate communication, and arrangements are made according to patients' personal preferences in accommodations, diet, and other needs.

Comprehensive Scope

Taiwan's medical system provides a wide range of services, from preventive healthcare to plastic surgery, dental surgery, weight control, sleep medicine, cardiac surgery, joint replacement, organ transplantation, and much more. Most hospitals in Taiwan offer health examination packages to serve each patient's unique needs, and treatments and recovery regimens often combine traditional Chinese medicine with Western medicine. The goal of this holistic approach is to integrate body, mind, and spirit for each patient's optimal health and well-being.

Affordability

In the course of developing a top-quality medical system for its own citizens, Taiwan has simultaneously achieved a level of affordability and efficiency that's attractive to international health travelers. Generally speaking, the surgical fees in Taiwan are about one-fifth to one-sixth of the prices patients are quoted in the US or the UK.

Notable Achievements

- 1978: World's fourth nation, and Asia's first, to achieve nation-wide hospital accreditation
- 1984: Asia's first successful liver transplant
- 1995: World's first endoscopic open-heart surgery
- 1995: Launch of the National Health Insurance (NHI) program, which achieved a 99 percent health insurance coverage rate for Taiwan's citizens by 2005
- 1996: Asia's first successful artificial heart transplant
- 1997: World's first living-donor liver transplant without blood transfusion
- 1998: World's first successful cardiac cryosurgery
- 1999: Asia's first microstereotactic deep-brain stimulation surgery for Parkinson's disease
- 2000: Asia's youngest-ever heart transplant patient

- 2001: Invention of potassium-hydrogen-phthalate (KHP) therapy, the treatment option with the highest cure rate for nasopharyngeal cancer (NPC)
- 2001: World's first successful skin stem cell treatment for corneal transplant
- 2003: Worldwide recognition for management of severe acute respiratory syndrome (SARS) epidemics
- 2003: World's first successful autologous stem cell transplant to treat NPC
- 2004: World's largest clinical trial of human papillovirus (HPV-008) vaccine for cervical cancer
- 2005: Asia's first successful positive cross-matched, living-donor kidney transplant
- 2006: World's first successful endoscopic potassium-titanyl-phosphate (KTP) laser surgery for recurrent NPC
- 2006: World's first pharmacogenomic testing to predict interferon therapy efficacy for treating patients with chronic hepatitis C

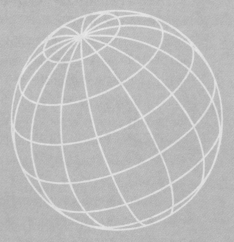

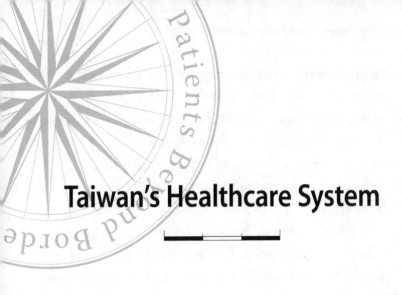

Taiwan's Healthcare System

According to a 2008 Department of Health (DOH) survey, Taiwan has 529 hospitals and 19,472 clinics. Thanks to Taiwan's nationwide accreditation system, the quality of personnel, facilities, instruments, and service in any hospital or clinic can be constantly maintained and enhanced. Accreditation levels vary. (See "The Hospital Accreditation System in Taiwan," below.) Those medical institutions with higher levels of accreditation have demonstrated that they can provide better medical services, and they receive higher rates of reimbursement from the Bureau of National Health Insurance (BNHI), a division of DOH.

National Health Insurance

To pursue social equity and meet the healthcare needs of the elderly and poor populations in Taiwan, BNHI launched the National Health Insurance (NHI) program in 1995. Enrollment in this government-run, single-payer program is mandatory for all citizens of Taiwan and for foreigners who reside in Taiwan for more than four months. NHI's mission is to provide universal coverage, low premiums, a comprehensive scope of benefits, easy access to medical treatment, proper care for disadvantaged groups, and a high level of public satisfaction.

Currently 99 percent of the Taiwanese people are enrolled in the NHI system, and more than 91 percent of Taiwan's healthcare providers are NHI-contracted medical institutions. By providing comprehensive healthcare coverage, NHI gives the citizens of Taiwan complete freedom to choose their preferred healthcare providers without the hassles of long queues and lengthy waiting periods. Under this program, all the people of Taiwan have nearly equal financial access to comprehensive health services, with protection against large medical expenses.

As a result of the NHI program, the total healthcare expenditure in Taiwan accounts for only 6 percent of the nation's gross domestic product (GDP). By comparison, healthcare spending in the US accounts for 15.3 percent of the GDP. In annual BNHI surveys, NHI is continually rated as Taiwan's most favored public program, with about 70 percent public satisfaction. This rating shows NHI has greatly improved the convenience, accessibility, and affordability of healthcare in Taiwan.

The Hospital Accreditation System in Taiwan

In 1968 the Ministry of Education, aiming to improve the training of medical students, developed the Hospital Accreditation Program to evaluate teaching hospitals. A decade later, with support from the Congress and Taiwan's health insurance authorities, the program was adopted by DOH and applied to all types of hospitals. Participation was voluntary, but the incentive was powerful: only accredited hospitals were allowed to provide healthcare through NHI. In 1999 a not-for-profit organization, the Taiwan Joint Commission on Hospital Accreditation (TJCHA), was established to manage the accreditation program. In 2006–2007 TJCHA became the first organization in Asia to be ISQua-certified for its operation as an accrediting body and also for the accreditation standards it developed.

Hospital accreditation has played a major role in the effort to promote quality healthcare in Taiwan. TJCHA's surveyors are drawn from a list of experts recommended by hospitals and organizations of health professionals. Surveyors must meet qualification requirements, take training courses, and attend a consensus workshop before conducting on-site surveys of hospitals. Once granted to a hospital, TJCHA accreditation is valid for three or four years. The accreditation program has demonstrated its efficacy in improving hospital services. For instance, it can be used to urge hospitals to demonstrate their commitment to patients or apply quality-surveillance tools and other measures, such as self-assessment and benchmark learning.

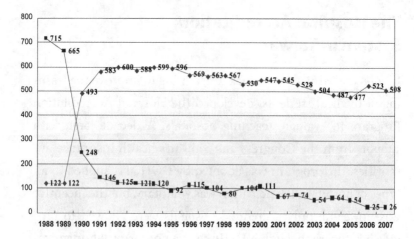

Figure 1. Number of Hospitals Surveyed by the TJCHA Hospital Accreditation Program 1988–2007

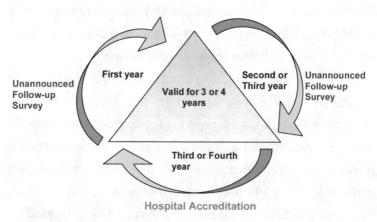

Figure 2. The Cycle of Hospital Accreditation

In 2003 Taiwan's Hospital Accreditation Program was re-formed to better embrace patient safety, patient-centered health-care, and community outreach. A new system was developed, tested, and adopted in 2005. To focus on the whole hospital instead of individual specialties, the new system divided on-site surveys into three domains: medicine, nursing, and administration. Standards were revised to better evaluate processes and outcomes. Measures were also devised to promote the skills of surveyors and to enhance the openness and fairness of the survey process.

The Taiwan Medicine Initiative: The Taiwan Task Force on Medical Travel (TTFMT)

Launched in 2007, TTFMT, which is administered by the Taiwan Nongovernmental Hospitals and Clinics Association, is a platform for integrating resources and encouraging cooperation across governmental organizations, related industries, and medical institutions. Supported by the Tourism Bureau, Government Information Office, Taiwan External Trade Development Council, Chung-Hua Institution for Economic Research, and DOH, TTFMT has brought 20 qualified hospitals into an alliance to promote to patients all over the world the five-star medical service that Taiwan can offer them.

The Tourism Bureau and the Government Information Office provide information about tourism and help promote Taiwan to the international media. The Taiwan External Trade Development Council communicates with overseas coadjutant organizations. The Chung-Hua Institution for Economic Research is responsible for the academic, field, and statistics research needed for TTFMT's marketing survey reports.

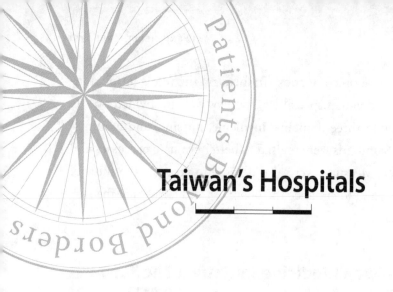

Taiwan's Hospitals

Buddhist Tzu Chi General Hospital

No. 707 Chung Yang Road, Section 3
Hualien 970, TAIWAN
Tel: 886 3 856.1825; 886 3 857.8600 (manual registration);
886 3 856.2016 (medical consultation)
Fax: 886 3 856.0977
Email: yilee@tzuchi.com.tw
Web: www.tzuchi.com.tw

Opened in August 1986, Buddhist Tzu Chi General Hospital was TJCHA-accredited as a Medical Center in 2002. ISO certification came that same year. Today, the hospital operates nearly 1,000 beds and employs more than 300 physicians and surgeons. The hospital's commitment to holistic medicine means that interdisciplinary methods of diagnosis and treatment are used with many patients.

Buddhist Tzu Chi General Hospital performs a wide range of procedures, from organ transplantation to laser cosmetic surgery and high-tech health screening. Other specialty areas include stroke treatment, stem cell research, malignant tumor treatment, and orthopedic surgery (especially total knee replacement, ankylosing spondylitis correction, and minimally invasive spinal surgery).

The hospital's numerous research centers include the **Neuro-Medical Scientific Center,** which provides a stereotactic navigation system for localization of brain vascular diseases and tumors and uses Gamma Knife radiosurgery for brain tumors. Surgeons in the **Department of Thoracic and Cardiovascular Surgery** perform coronary artery bypass grafting (CABG), off-pump (beating-heart) CABG, peripheral artery bypass grafting, lung cancer surgery, esophageal reconstruction, esophageal varices repair, video-assisted thoracoscopic surgery, balloon angioplasty, stenting, and more. Noninvasive procedures for diagnosis and management include echocardiography, treadmill electrocardiogram (ECG) testing, and 24-hour ambulatory ECG recording.

The **Voiding Dysfunctional Center under the Department of Urology** has achieved international standards in both research and clinical medicine, continuing to develop new cures for voiding-dysfunctional patients. Diagnostic and therapeutic methods include renal sonography, video examination, and endoscopic surgery when necessary.

The **Stem Cell Center,** a bone marrow registry to assist people with blood diseases, was established in 1993. More than 280,000 donors are now registered. In its 15 years of operation, the center has helped find donors for more than 1,000 patients in 23 countries.

Specialties

✦ Cardiology

✦ Thoracic and cardiovascular surgery

✦ Organ transplantation

✦ Orthopedic surgery

✦ Cancer prevention

✦ Deep-brain stimulation surgery (for Parkinson's disease)

✦ Voiding dysfunction surgery

✦ Bone marrow transplantation

✦ High-tech health checkups

✦ Laser surgery

Services Provided for International Patients

✦ Free pickup service from Hualien Airport or Hualien Railway Station

✦ Arrangements for meals and accommodations

✦ Sightseeing tours

Achievements

✦ 1999: National Innovation Award Taiwan, to the Hospice Care Team

✦ 2002: National Innovation Award Taiwan, for the United U2 Hip System

✦ 2006: National Innovation Award Taiwan, for the Ostomy Drainable Pouch

Feature Story

Tzu Chi Goes International

Tzu Chi International Medical Association began spreading the seeds of compassion around the world in 2003, starting with the successful separation of conjoined twins from the Philippines. After hours of complicated surgery at Buddhist Tzu Chi General Hospital, Lea and Rachel were finally able to have independent lives.

In the summer of 2004, a five-year-old boy named Novemthree came to Buddhist Tzu Chi General Hospital from Batam, Indonesia. He had gigantiform cementoma, a massive, heavy tumor that covered his face and severely altered his facial features. After five difficult and complex operations, the boy was able to smile once again. This "mission impossible" accomplishment earned high praise for the medical team from specialists at the Mayo Clinic (US).

In 2004 the Pan siblings from Singapore, Jing-yang and Zi-qi, underwent treatment for Hallervorden-Spatz syndrome, an inherited disorder of the brain and nervous system. With the application of deep-brain stimulation and daily physical therapy at Tzu Chi, in just half a year Jing-yang was able to use his legs to walk, and Zi-qi greatly improved her ability to walk without assistance.

Cathay General Hospital

280 Jen-Ai Road, Section 4
Taipei 106, TAIWAN
Tel: 886 2 2708.2121 ext. 1312
Fax: 886 2 2708.2430
Email: isc@cgh.org.tw
Web: www1.cgh.org.tw/index.htm

Located in the center of Taipei City, Cathay General Hospital was founded in 1977 by Cathay Life Insurance, a subsidiary of the Lin-Yuan Group. Its main specialty is the treatment of heart disease and related disorders through its **Institute of Cardiovascular Medicine.** To diagnose and treat heart conditions, Cathay has invested in the latest medical imaging equipment, such as a Gemini GXL positron emission tomography/computed tomography (PET/CT) scanner, a 1.5-Tesla magnetic resonance imaging (MRI) scanner, and a 64-multidetector CT scanner. Because prevention is key, Cathay has organized a comprehensive general health examination department with a highly qualified professional staff, many of whom are fluent in English or other languages.

Specialties

✦ Cardiovascular: acute coronary syndrome, congestive heart failure, cardiac arrhythmia, valvular heart disease, congenital heart disease, preventive cardiology, cardiomyopathy, peripheral vessel disease, percutaneous coronary intervention

✦ Orthopedic: total hip replacement, total knee replacement

Services Provided for International Patients

✦ Arrangements for accommodations

✦ Airport pickup and transportation

✦ Assistance before, during, and after hospitalization

✦ Direct admission arrangements

✦ Flight reservations and confirmation

✦ Language translation

✦ Medical referrals

✦ Scheduling of appointments

✦ Customer-oriented medical services

✦ Separate facilities for sick and well clients

✦ Interprofessional consultation with rapid resolution

✦ Escorts to medical appointments and procedures

Achievements

✦ 2004, 2005: Patents for placental stem cell transformation into nerve cells and successful culturing of amniotic fluid derived from mesenchymal stem cells

✦ 2005: Taiwan Joint Commission on Hospital Accreditation (TJCHA) accreditation as a Medical Center (the first-class level of hospital in Taiwan)

✦ 2006: Sixth-place ranking among the top 500 organizations in the medical and social services industry in *Common Wealth* magazine

✦ 2006: Third-place ranking among Taiwan's medical centers in a *Global View* magazine survey

Feature Story

The 280-Minute CPR Miracle

In December 2005, Miss Chen, a 28-year-old dancer, developed an acute isolated viral myocarditis (inflammation of the membrane around the heart). Upon her admission to Cathay General Hospital, her condition was diagnosed as serious and she was sent to the intensive care unit immediately.

That night, when the on-duty cardiologist, Dr. Yeh, made his 6 o'clock rounds, Miss Chen was asking for McDonald's food — but just a few minutes later, her heart suddenly stopped beating, and her condition quickly deteriorated.

Dr. Yeh immediately began performing cardiopulmonary resuscitation (CPR) on Miss Chen and arranged for her transfer to National Taiwan University Hospital (NTUH), which has an artificial heart-lung machine that provides extracorporeal membrane oxygenation (ECMO) for life support. On the way to NTUH by ambulance, Dr. Yeh single-handedly performed CPR for 60 minutes.

At NTUH, the primary cardiologist found that, despite their efforts, Miss Chen could not be connected to ECMO because she was too thin and had been given too much heart stimulant before arriving at the hospital. Furthermore, intubation was not possible because her vessels were too small.

As nurses and doctors continued to perform CPR, Miss Chen was moved to the operating room, where a thoracotomy (opening of the chest) was performed until the ECMO could run normally. After 200 minutes of CPR at NTUH, Miss Chen was successfully resuscitated.

This total resuscitation time of 280 minutes holds the world's record as the longest successful CPR—and even doctors call this a miracle.

Chang Gung Memorial Hospital

Chang Gung Memorial Hospital–Linkou Branch
No. 5 Fu Hsing Street
Gueishan Township, Taoyuan, TAIWAN

Chang Gung Memorial Hospital–Taipei Branch
No. 199 Tung Hwa North Road
Taipei, TAIWAN

Chang Gung Memorial Hospital–Taoyuan Branch
No. 123 Dinghu Road
Jioulu Village, Gueishan Township, Taoyuan, TAIWAN

Chang Gung Memorial Hospital–Kaohsiung Branch
No. 123 Taipei Road
Niao Sung Hsiang, Kaohsiung, TAIWAN

International Service Center of CGMH
Tel: 886 3 319.6200 ext. 2555
Fax: 886 3 319.8001
Email: isc@cgmh.org.tw
Web: www.cgmh.org.tw

Chang Gung Memorial Hospital (CGMH) was founded in 1976 as a nonprofit hospital and is part of a larger healthcare network that includes Chang Gung University, Chang Gung Institute of Nursing, acute hospitals, chronic hospitals, and the Chang

Gung Nursing Home and Aging Village. Administrators say that among the citizens of Taiwan, one in every seven chooses to visit one of the hospitals in the Chang Gung network for medical care.

Overall, nearly 13,000 people work in the Chang Gung network. Its 2,500 physicians and surgeons serve patients occupying almost 9,000 beds. The Chang Gung network stresses medical research and education as well as clinical services. CGMH has become a training center for doctors from Europe, the US, and Southeast Asia.

To provide overseas clients with better services, CGMH has established an **International Service Center.** Its staff members help with appointments, treatment planning, travel planning, and cost estimates. Some 500 international patients seek treatment at Chang Gung annually.

CGMH's specialty centers include a **Craniofacial Center, Aesthetic Medical Center, Liver Transplant Center, Reconstructive Microsurgery Center, Joint Replacement Center, Hematopoietic Stem Cell Transplantation Center, Cardiovascular Center, Implant Center, Voice Beauty Center,** and **Healthcare Center.**

Specialties

✦ Craniomaxillofacial deformity: more than 800 remedied annually (e.g., orofacial cleft, secondary cleft deformity, complex craniofacial deformity)

✦ Dermatology and plastic surgery (including well-rounded beauty and fitness consultation)

✦ Liver transplant: more than 500, with one of the highest patient survival rates in the world

✦ Reconstructive microsurgery: created numerous world-renowned surgical techniques, such as replantation and brachial plexus reconstruction

✦ Joint replacement: 1,500 annually

✦ Hematopoietic stem cell transplant: 85 percent success rate of umbilical cord–blood transplant for critical anemia, acute leukemia, osteoporosis, and aplastic anemia

✦ Carotid artery stenting: 99 percent success rate, complication rate less than 1 percent

✦ Dental implants: more than 1,000 annually

✦ Treatment of complicated voice disorders including unilateral vocal palsy, vocal atrophy, vocal deficit, spasmodic dysphonia, and androphonia, as well as pitch elevation surgery (for male-to-female transgender patients) (About 800 operations have been performed since the center's establishment in 2003, with a patient-satisfaction rating exceeding 90 percent.)

✦ Checkups and preventive medicine: whole-body health, positron emission tomography/computed tomography (PET/CT) cancer check, advanced cardiovascular examination with high-speed CT, advanced nervous system examination with magnetic resonance imaging (MRI)

Services Provided for International Patients

✦ Assistance with making physician appointments

✦ Assistance with mapping out the medical treatment plan

✦ Troubleshooting for visa applications

✦ Transportation and accommodation arrangements

✦ Language services, including English and Chinese

✦ Preparation of medical treatment itinerary for overseas clients

✦ Accompaniment service: hospital orientation and guidance through the whole medical process

✦ Daily visit service

✦ Discharge service

Achievements

✦ 1988–2008: TJCHA accreditation of Linkou, Taipei, and Kaohsiung Branches as Medical Centers

✦ 1984: Asia's first successful liver transplant

✦ 1995: World's first endoscopic open-heart surgery

✦ 1995: Number one on list of most-admired institutes in health-care, *The Common Wealth*

✦ 1997: World's first living-donor liver transplant without blood transfusion

✦ 2003: Taiwan's first College of American Pathologists (CAP) accreditation

✦ 2007 – 2008: Number one on list of trusted brands, annual *Reader's Digest* customers' reliability survey

Feature Story

Surgery Lets Boy Eat Steak

December 1, 2001, was a miraculous day for Kevin, a 16-year-old boy from the island of Mauritius off the African coast. On that day, he underwent an orthognathic surgery in Taiwan that changed his life forever.

Kevin was born with craniofacial deformities that prevented him from speaking clearly, and he sometimes had difficulty breathing because his tongue clogged his airways. Before he came to Taiwan, Kevin had undergone several plastic and reconstructive surgeries, which had partially improved his facial appearance, but he still needed advanced reconstructive procedures to significantly improve his facial structure and his bite. He couldn't chew hard food; he could eat only liquid and soft foods. Kevin's mother said her son dreamed of eating a steak someday.

Initially, Kevin's family had planned to take him to South Africa for the surgery. However, Dr. Ian Munro, a leading craniofacial surgeon, recommended that Kevin visit his former student, Dr. Yu-Ray Chen, now the superintendent of Chang Gung Memorial Hospital (CGMH) in Taiwan. Kevin and his family took Dr. Munro's advice and flew 11 hours to make their dream come true.

CGMH arranged a professional team, including the hospital's chief surgeon, Dr. Yu-Ray Chen, and craniofacial dental surgeon, Dr. Jiong-Xing Huang, to perform the complicated procedure. The surgery extended the maxilla (upper jaw) forward by 2 centimeters and pushed the mandible (lower jaw) back by 1 centimeter to make the jawbones fit together properly. A piece of Kevin's rib that measured about 11 centimeters (about 4 inches) was used to fill gaps in the jawbones.

After the successful surgery, Kevin could easily close his mouth, a feat he had never before been able to accomplish—and one month after the procedure, Kevin tasted steak for the first time in his life.

Changhua Christian Hospital

No. 135 Nansiao Street
Changhua City, Changhua 500, TAIWAN
Tel: 886 4 728.5161 (International Clinic hotline)
Fax: 886 4 723.2942
Email: imsc@mail.cch.org.tw
Web: www2.cch.org.tw

In operation since 1896, Changhua Christian Hospital (CCH) has 1,366 beds and more than 550 surgeons and physicians. The hospital aims to "uphold the Bible as its moral standard, Christian faith as its foundation, patient safety as its priority, and health for all as its goal."

CCH offers a full range of specialty departments, including internal medicine, surgery, neurology, dermatology, radiation oncology, otolaryngology, ophthalmology, oncology, gastroenterology, genetic counseling, medical imaging, nuclear medicine, dentistry, and pediatrics. It was accredited as a Medical Center by TJCHA in 2000. Its first kidney transplant and its first liver transplant took place in 2001. The CCH Institutional Review Board closely oversees patients' interests and safety.

Specialties

✦ Gynecology

✦ Oncology

✦ Reproductive medicine

✦ Neurology

✦ Chinese medicine

✦ Orthopedic surgery

✦ Minimally invasive surgery

✦ Living-donor transplantation

✦ Joint reconstruction

Services Provided for International Patients

✦ English information hotline

✦ Medical appointment scheduling

✦ Language and document translation

✦ Airport pickup

✦ Assistance before and after hospitalization

✦ Discharge planning

✦ Medical referrals

✦ Day-tour information

✦ Flight reservations and confirmations

✦ Visa extensions

Achievements

✦ 2005: The Asia-Pacific territory's first certification of an Institutional Review Board by the WHO Forum for Ethical Review Committees in Asia and the Western Pacific Region

✦ 2005: First-place ranking for courtesy in ambulatory service in *Common Health* magazine

✦ 2005: *Common Health* magazine Award for Excellence in Medical Informational Service

✦ 2006: Executive Yuan Research, Development, and Evaluation Commission Award for Excellence in Fostering an English-Compatible Environment

✦ 2007: Bilingual Outstanding Genial Hospital Award by DOH and TCHE: Promoting Bilingual Environment for Hospital

Feature Story

Brain Surgery for an HIV Patient

Miss Lin, a volunteer at the Tzu-Chi Elementary School in northern Thailand, had been suffering from headaches. She had a computed tomography (CT) scan at a hospital in Taipei and was diagnosed with a brain tumor. Before receiving any further medical treatment, Miss Lin revealed to her doctors that she was infected with human immunodeficiency virus (HIV). Her condition had caused some medical institutions to refuse their services because of the risk of infection.

Shu-Mei Chiou, the administrator of the Garden of Mercy Foundation, contacted Changhua Christian Hospital. The Changhua staff believes that everyone should have equal access to medical treatment, so they decided to help Miss Lin. Because her condition was known in advance, the hospital enacted exacting procedures to prevent any transmission of the virus during her surgery. Miss Lin's tumor was successfully removed, and she is now working again at the school in Thailand.

China Medical University Hospital

No. 2 Yuh-Der Road
Taichung City 40447, TAIWAN
Tel: 886 4 2205.2121
Fax: 886 4 2203.8303
Email: imc@mail.cmuh.org.tw
Web: ims.cmuh.org.tw

China Medical University Hospital (CMUH), the first hospital in Taiwan to integrate Chinese and Western medicine, was established in 1980. Its eight comprehensive centers are a **Stroke Center, Cancer Center, Trauma and Emergency Center, Heart and Vascular Center, Organ Transplantation Center, Neuropsychiatry Center, Kidney Institute,** and **Preventive Medicine Center.** Each attending physician holds a certification in a Western medical specialty; most also have subspecialties. All CMUH physicians have received both Chinese and Western clinical training. More than 1,000 registered nurses provide not only basic clinical care but also sophisticated care in the intensive care unit, emergency room, and specialty centers.

The development of medical services for international patients has become a priority at CMUH in recent years. That mission is supported by academic exchange and cooperative agreements with the University of South Carolina (US), MD Anderson Cancer Center at the University of Texas (US), and Policlinico San Matteo – University Pavia (Italy).

Specialties

✦ Chinese medicine

✦ Cardiology

✦ Cardiothoracic vascular surgery

✦ Plastic surgery

✦ Joint replacement surgery with Chinese rehabilitation

✦ Percutaneous coronary intervention

✦ Organ transplantation

✦ Stroke treatment

✦ Ophthalmology

✦ Laser treatment

✦ Rehabilitation

✦ Sports medicine

✦ Hemodialysis and peritoneal dialysis

Services Provided for International Patients

+ Transportation

+ Hotel or long-term lodging arrangements for patients and families

+ Air ambulance services

+ Assistance before, during, and after hospitalization

+ Interpretation services in English, Japanese, and Arabic

+ Translation of medical documents

+ Discharge planning

+ Health examinations for patient's families

+ Special foods and nutrition services

+ Followup care

+ Communications assistance, including calling, faxing, and Internet

+ Shopping, sightseeing, and travel planning

Achievements

+ 2001: IV National Biotechnology Medical Quality Award, Community Service Quality Award, and Specialty Medical Quality Award in the Department of Community Medicine and Pharmacology

✦ 2002: The Department of Medical Genetics received the Golden Award in National Biotech and Medicine

✦ 2004: Accredited by the Department of Health and the Ministry of Education as a Medical Center

✦ 2005: National Biotechnology and Medical Care Quality Award to the Department of Neonatology

✦ 2007: Participated in International Cooperation and Development Fund (ICDF) Mobile Medical Mission to St. Kitts and Nevis

✦ 2007: Established Cancer Center and Critical Care Center

Feature Story

Boy Receives Bone Marrow Transplant

Sudan in North Africa was unfamiliar to China Medical University Hospital (CMUH) staff until Omar, a cute little Sudanese boy, arrived for bone marrow transplantation. Omar had been diagnosed with Fanconi anemia, a rare genetic disease that interferes with bone marrow growth and often causes leukemia; patients may also develop other cancers and limb deformities. Unfortunately, Omar was not the only child in his family to be afflicted. One of his brothers passed away due to Fanconi anemia, and his other brother, Enour, also has it. Two other brothers are unaffected.

Omar's family faced insurmountable financial obstacles in obtaining the necessary medical treatment until Mrs. Tsai, whose Sudanese husband works in the trade business between Taiwan and Sudan, heard about the family's situation in 2003 when visiting her family in

Sudan. Mrs. Tsai inquired for help at all of the medical centers in Taiwan. When CMUH decided to treat Omar with stem cell transplantation, the hospital opened a foundation account so people could help Omar's two healthy brothers come to Taiwan to serve as donors.

Omar's stem cell transplant was successfully completed in January 2007. CMUH held a party to celebrate Omar's birthday on July 1 of that year, and Omar popped a balloon to symbolize his defeat of his illness. CMUH is still fundraising for Enour's treatment.

E-Da Hospital

No. 1 Jiau-Shu Tsuen Road, Yan-Chao Shiang
Kaohsiung County 824, TAIWAN
Tel: 886 7 615.0011 ext. 5760
Fax: 886 7 615.5352
Email: ed103221@edah.org.tw
Web: www.edah.org.tw

E-Da Hospital opened its doors in 2004. The 230 physicians and surgeons of this teaching hospital treat patients in a 1,122-bed facility that boasts impressive modern architecture and luxurious interior decor, complete with pianists performing in the lobby, light and water shows, art exhibits, and numerous cultural activities.

E-Da's doctors specialize in minimally invasive surgery, esophageal and voice reconstruction, total joint replacement, brachial plexus injury, hyperhidrosis (excessive sweating), Gamma Knife radiosurgery, prostate laser surgery, sleep assessment, and cardiac catheterization. E-Da employs technologically advanced equipment, including positron emission tomography/computed tomography (PET/CT), 64-slice CT, and magnetic resonance imaging (MRI). Surgeons performed E-Da's first liver and kidney transplants in 2006.

Dr. Chin-Kun Huang, chief of the **International Endoscopic Obesity Center** at E-Da, performs mostly gastric bypass operations, with smaller numbers of LAP-BAND and sleeve gastrectomies. He is a member of the Asia-Pacific Bariatric Surgery Society and the International Federation for the Surgery of Obesity.

Specialties

✦ Plastic surgery: esophageal and voice reconstruction, lymphedema treatment, laser treatment

✦ Neurosurgery: hyperhidrosis treatment, spinal fusion, discectomy, Gamma Knife radiosurgery

✦ Orthopedics: total knee replacement, total hip replacement, treatment of brachial plexus injury

✦ General surgery: laparoscopic bariatric surgery, liver transplant

✦ Urology: prostate laser surgery, kidney transplant

✦ Cardiology: cardiac catheterization examination with intervention

✦ Cardiovascular surgery: coronary artery bypass graft (CABG), valve replacement

✦ Obstetrics and gynecology: laparoscopic surgery, hysteroscopic surgery

✦ Neurology: polysomnography

✦ Bariatric surgery: LAP-BAND, gastric bypass

✦ Dentistry: tooth whitening, ceramic veneers

✦ Physical examinations (Health Examination Center)

✦ Cancer diagnosis and treatment: PET/CT, whole-body tumor survey

✦ CT and MRI: coronary CT; low-radiation chest CT, brain CT, and brain MRI; cerebral and neck MRI

Services Provided for International Patients

✦ Assistance with visa applications and extensions

✦ Arrangements for accommodations

✦ Airport pickup

✦ Arrangements for local transportation

✦ Direct admission

✦ International ward

✦ Language translation

✦ Arrangements for excursions

✦ Post-surgery followup through Web conference

Achievements

✦ 2004: TJCHA accreditation as a Regional Teaching Hospital

✦ 2006: ISO 15189: 2007 Certification

✦ 2007: Taiwan's first chromatin remodeling application, producing a hairless guinea pig

✦ 2007: Bilingual Genial Hospital Award by DOH and TCHE: Promoting Bilingual Environment for Hospital

✦ 2008: TJCHA accreditation as a Hospital and a Teaching Hospital

Feature Story

New Life for an Obese Patient

Joe, an American citizen and English professor, was working in Taiwan when he first contacted Dr. Huang at E-Da Hospital. Joe weighed 170 kilograms (about 375 pounds), making him a super-obese patient. Obesity had led to many diseases for Joe, including diabetes mellitus, hypertension, cardiac disease, obstructive sleep apnea, and varicose veins in his lower extremities. He was taking ten different medications for multiple medical problems and had developed a "duck-walk" due to severe degenerative changes in his knee joints.

When Dr. Huang reviewed his patient's medical history, he found that, two years before, Joe had experienced a sudden-onset cardiac and respiratory arrest that nearly killed him. In a single year, Joe had been admitted to the hospital five times. Although Joe was well aware of his obesity-related diseases and had tried various methods to lose weight, he always regained the weight. Dr. Huang realized that Joe might die soon without treatment for his obesity.

Dr. Huang treated Joe with laparoscopic Roux-en-Y gastric bypass surgery, a procedure that reduces stomach size and limits the amount of food the patient can consume. Joe recovered quickly and was discharged seven days after surgery. Three months later, his weight was down to 125 kg (about 275 pounds), and his blood pressure and blood sugar were normal without the need to control them with drugs. He also no longer needed to wear a continuous positive airway pressure (CPAP) mask to keep his upper airway open during sleep. Today Joe's weight is 75 kg (about 165 pounds).

Kaohsiung Medical University Chung-Ho Memorial Hospital

No. 100, Tzyou First Road
Kaohsiung City 807, TAIWAN
Tel: 886 7 312.1101 ext. 5500
Fax: 886 7 320.8298
Email: 960542@ms.kmuh.org.tw
Web: www.kmuh.org.tw

Kaohsiung Medical University Chung-Ho Memorial Hospital (KMUH), established in 1957, is a multispecialty hospital located in Kaohsiung City. It is one of the largest hospitals in southern Taiwan, with 1,600 beds and eight specialty centers, including craniofacial reconstruction, total joint replacement, cardiovascular intervention, cardiac surgery, and dental implantation.

In 1978 KMUH was one of the first four hospitals accredited by TJCHA as a First-Class Teaching Hospital. Since then, KMUH has expanded its facilities and purchased the latest in medical equipment, including a 3-Tesla magnetic resonance imaging (MRI) scanner and a 64-slice computed tomography (CT) scanner. The hospital also uses positron emission tomography (PET) and provides TomoTherapy radiation treatments. The **Kao-Xing Center for International Medical Service** serves the needs of health travelers.

Specialties

✦ Cardiovascular intervention and cardiac surgery

✦ Craniofacial surgery

✦ Total knee and total hip arthroplasty

✦ Odontectomy (including extraction of impacted teeth)

✦ Cosmetic dentistry: power-bleaching, stain removal, porcelain veneers

✦ Removable denture construction

✦ Dental implant therapy

✦ Body contour surgery

✦ Facial cosmetic surgery

✦ Endoscope-assisted correction of primary varicose veins

✦ Chinese internal medicine

✦ Health examinations using high-quality equipment

Services Provided for International Patients

✦ Airport pickup and transportation

✦ Arrangements for accommodations

✦ Assistance before, during, and after hospitalization

✦ Direct admission arrangements

✦ Flight reservations and confirmations

✦ Language translation

✦ Medical referrals

✦ Scheduling of appointments

✦ Visa extensions

Achievements

✦ 2005: TJCHA Healthcare Quality Improvement Circle Awards for improving outpatients' time between making an appointment and visiting, improving the noise of ICU in neurosurgery, and improving inpatients' oral hygiene in the psychiatric department

✦ 2006: Symbol of National Quality, Surgical Skill Center

✦ 2007: Symbol of National Quality, Integrated Chronic Kidney Disease Care Program, and Leader of Chronic Kidney Disease Care in Taiwan

✦ 2007: British Standards Institution Certification

✤ 2007: ISO 27001 Certification

✤ 2007: Information Security Management System (ISMS) Certification

Lotung Poh-Ai Hospital

Lo-Hsu Foundation, Inc.
No. 83 Nan Chang Street, Lotung Division
Yilan County 265, TAIWAN
Tel: 886 3 954.3131
Fax: 886 3 954.5555
Email: 96a014@mail.pohai.org.tw
Web: www.pohai.org.tw

Lotung Poh-Ai Hospital (LPA) opened in 1953 as a 30-bed, small-scale general hospital. Originally a hospital for Yilan County residents, LPA is now a teaching hospital with 1,100 beds and 140 physicians practicing 36 medical specialties. It is an acute- and intensive-care, community-focused medical center and a tertiary medical referral center for Yilan County.

LPA is affiliated with National Taiwan University Hospital, Taipei Veterans General Hospital, Buddhist Tzu Chi General Hospital, Shin Kong Wu Ho-Su Memorial Hospital, Cheng Hsin Rehabilitation Medical Center, National Yang-Ming University, and China Medical University. Its major specialties include neurosurgery, cardiology, cardiovascular surgery, orthopedics, and cosmetic medicine. LPA's orthopedics department handles approximately 3,000 cases every year. The hospital's facilities for minimally invasive surgery have been operating since 2007.

LPA's **Medical Center of Oncology** was established in 2002 and is headed by a specialist in liver cancer. Physicians at the hospital's **Neuroscience Medical Center,** established in 2003, use the latest three-band radiofrequency thermocoagulator to treat neuropathic and intractable pain.

Specialties

✦ Orthopedics: fracture surgery, arthroscopic surgery, spine surgery, total joint reconstruction (arthroplasty), limb removal, hand surgery, minimally invasive surgery, orthopedic trauma, spine surgery, sports medicine, hand surgery

✦ Cardiology: cardiothoracic and vascular surgery, balloon dilatation or stent placement for acute myocardial blade, balloon catheter, intravascular stent, intravascular ultrasound, open-heart surgery, peripheral vascular bypass surgery

Services Provided for International Patients

✦ Scheduling of appointments

✦ Ample time for clinical visit to allow for detailed discussion with the physician and appropriate treatments

✦ Medical referrals

✦ Arrangements for accommodations

✦ Airport pickup and transportation

✦ Assistance before, during, and after hospitalization

✦ Flight reservations and confirmations

✦ Language translation

Achievements

✦ 2006: TJCHA New Hospital Accreditation as an Excellent Teaching Hospital

✦ 2006: ISO 15189: 2003 Certification

✦ 2006: Taiwan Accreditation Foundation–Chinese National Laboratory Accreditation (TAF–CNLA) Certification of Laboratory Medicine

✦ 2006: Taiwan Academy of Physical Medicine and Rehabilitation Certification

✦ 2006: Taiwan Otolaryngological Society Certification

✦ 2006: Taiwan Society of Pulmonary and Critical Care Medicine Certification

✦ 2007: Taiwan Society of Internal Medicine Certification

✦ 2007: Taiwan Surgical Association Certification

✦ 2007: Taiwan Neurological Society Certification

✦ 2007: Taiwan Urological Association Certification

Feature Story

Brain Tumor Surgery on an 82-Year-Old Grandmother

Over a period of five years, Mrs. Wu, an 82-year-old grandmother, had experienced gradual loss of mobility in her left leg and arm. Her family originally attributed her decline to an artificial knee-joint implant, but after a detailed checkup by Dr. Hsing-Hong Chen, the superintendent of Lotung Poh-Ai Hospital, and his medical team, the cause was found to be a pituitary gland tumor pressing on the surrounding nerves.

After consultation by the superintendent and his medical team with family members, the decision was made to remove the tumor surgically. After ten hours of microsurgery, Mrs. Wu regained normal function on the left side of her body. Mrs. Wu and her family expressed gratitude for the help and thoughtfulness of Dr. Chen and the surgeons at Lotung Poh-Ai Hospital.

Min-Sheng General Hospital

No. 168 Ching-Kuo Road, 22F
Taoyuan City 330, TAIWAN
Tel: 886 3 317.9599 ext. 2222 (24-hour hotline)
Fax: 886 3 346.3764 (Attn. International Health Care)
Email: missioncare.tw@gmail.com
Web: www.missioncare.com.tw

Established in 2001, Min-Sheng General Hospital has more than 600 beds and 120 physicians and surgeons. Min-Sheng staff members pride themselves on seamless care and one-on-one services to patients. The hospital's **International Health Care**

Center boasts "selective, low-risk, highly competitive health services and packages" — some of them set up to work with US health insurance plans. Such packages include coronary artery bypass graft (CABG), percutaneous transluminal coronary angioplasty (PTCA), cardiac catheterization, total knee replacement, total hip replacement, LASIK eye surgery, hernia repair, weight-loss surgery, colporrhaphy (surgical repair of a defect in the vaginal wall), vaginal hysterectomy, liposuction, tummy tuck, breast augmentation or reduction, and laminectomy (a spinal surgery for relieving back pain).

Min-Sheng also accepts overseas patients who need dialysis while traveling in Taiwan. The **Dialysis Center** is equipped with an online clearance monitor and single-use hollow fibers to assure adequacy and high quality.

While Min-Sheng has been serving its local patients for more than 30 years, its international services have expanded since its JCI accreditation in 2006. Min-Sheng's specialty centers focus on nephrology, emergency and acute care, digital imaging and digitally guided surgery, oncology, three-dimensional stereotactic scanning, sleep medicine, and 64-slice computed tomography (CT) scanning, among others.

Specialties

✦ Cardiovascular care (including mini-bypass cardiac surgery)

✦ Minimally invasive surgery (including bariatric)

✦ Orthopedic surgery: hip, knee, spine

✦ Women's and children's care

✦ Fertility and reproduction: in vitro fertilization (IVF)

✦ Health promotion and disease prevention (including comprehensive health checkup and VIP Health Screening)

✦ Cosmetic and plastic surgery

✦ LASIK vision correction

Services Provided for International Patients

✦ Customized service packages

✦ Installment payment plan available

✦ Airport pickup and taxi service

✦ English-speaking staff

✦ Transportation arrangements

✦ Minimal waiting

✦ Assistance with tour planning

✦ Hotel-like accommodations

✦ Preferred doctors

✦ Assistance in completing insurance claims

✦ Internet access to personal medical records

✦ Post-discharge followup contact

✦ 1:1 service for international patients

Achievements

✦ 2004: Asia's first *e-Speed* electron beam tomography (EBT) exam (lower radiation exposure than regular CT)

✦ 2005–2008: Ministry of Education: Certified as a Teaching Hospital for internal medicine, surgery, obstetrics and gynecology, pediatrics, orthopedics, and family medicine

✦ 2006–2009: ISO 9001: 2000 Certification (Provision of Laboratory Medicine Service)

✦ 2006–2009: ISO 15189: 2003 Certification (Department of Laboratory)

✦ 2006: Asia's first overseas telecast of live bariatric surgery

✦ 2007: Taiwan's first bioenteric intragastric balloon surgery

✦ 2007: Recognition for shorter "door to balloon" time than the international standard for cardiac catheterization by the *New England Journal of Medicine*

✦ 2007: Taiwan's first mobile extracorporeal membrane oxygenation (ECMO) ambulance

✦ Higher than 95 percent customer satisfaction rate and 80 percent customer return rate for the Executive Health Checkup Center

Feature Story

Couple Gains Family from Min-Sheng Hospital's Weight-Reduction Surgery

Stephen and Susan knew that bariatric surgery could help with their weight problems — but they did not realize how much it would change their lives.

Stephen is 32 years old and lives in Taichung. For business reasons, he frequently drives to Taipei or Taoyuan and returns the same day. The long drives and lack of exercise fueled his weight gain. His weight reached 107 kilograms (about 235 pounds) with a body mass index (BMI) as high as 36 (the normal BMI range is 18 – 25). Hoping to improve his health, Stephen decided to consider weight-reduction surgery, and he conducted extensive Internet research. He studied patients' experiences and media reports and even found out about the types of surgical equipment needed for these procedures.

Finally, in 2005, Steven decided to have endoscopic gastric bypass surgery at Min-Sheng General Hospital. The surgery was performed by Dr. Wei-Jei Lee, a leader in surgical weight reduction in the Asia-Pacific territory, who has performed over 1,900 weight-reduction surgeries.

Meanwhile Susan, from Taipei, had been limited by her weight problems for years. Her weight reached 95 kg (about 210 pounds) and her BMI value reached 38. This made her day-to-day life and work difficult, and she had not been able to attract a boyfriend. She tried many different methods to lose weight, but none had been successful. In 2006 Susan chose Min-Sheng to receive weight-loss surgery and start a different life. When she returned to the hospital for aftercare, she met Stephen. Similar surgery and recovery circumstances became their favorite topic of conversation and fostered the growth of their romantic relationship.

As Stephen's and Susan's life-long healthcare partner, Min-Sheng General Hospital continues to provide support and instruction after their surgeries. Both of them attended post-operative followups for a year. Stephen's weight has decreased to 75 kg (165 pounds) and Susan's has dropped to 60 kg (132 pounds). Their health has greatly improved and their lives have changed dramatically for the better. In May 2007, surrounded by family and friends, including Dr. Lee, Stephen and Susan married. The couple became parents in 2008.

National Cheng Kung University Hospital

No. 138 Sheng Li Road
Tainan City 70403, TAIWAN
Tel: 886 6 235.3535 ext. 4520
Fax: 886 6 236.9602
Email: ims@mail.hosp.ncku.edu.tw
Web: webpage.hosp.ncku.edu.tw/ims

Located in the northern district of Tainan City, National Cheng Kung University Hospital (NCKUH) opened in 1988. It is the only national university hospital and referral center in southern Taiwan and is DOH-accredited as a Medical Center. NCKUH staff provide medical, educational, and research services in 40 departments and six centers for emergent, critical, complicated, and rare diseases.

NCKUH has approximately 1,200 beds and 2,700 staff. Nearly 60 percent of its attending physicians are faculty members in the university's College of Medicine. Areas of specialization include minimally invasive joint replacement surgery, cardiovascular surgery and treatment, craniofacial and plastic surgery, health exams, tumor treatment, reproduction/infertility, and more.

Specialties

✦ Joint replacement surgery

✦ Cardiovascular interventional therapy and surgery

✦ Craniofacial and plastic surgery

✦ Cosmetic laser treatment

✦ Health examination

✦ Positron emission tomography/computed tomography (PET/CT) scanning

✦ Tumor treatment (image-guided radiotherapy)

✦ Assisted reproductive technology (ART)

Services Provided for International Patients

✦ A case coordinator to organize medical appointments

✦ Rapid arrangement of examinations and review of test results

✦ Professional pharmacists who explain prescription drugs in English

✦ Arrangement of admission and outpatient services

✦ Assistance with applying for medical certifications, such as proof of payment and copies of redical records

✦ Consultation on treatment plans

✦ Followup to check patient progress

Achievements

✦ 2004: National Biotechnology and Medical Care Quality Gold Award

✦ 2004: Symbol of National Quality, Developmental Care for Premature Infants

✦ 2005: National Biotechnology and Medical Care Quality Silver Award

✦ 2005: Symbol of National Quality, Hospice Palliative Care

✦ 2007: Executive Yuan Service Quality Award

✦ 2007: 18th National Quality Award (the highest national honor granted for the overall quality of a medical environment)

Feature Story

ABO-Incompatible Living-Donor Kidney Transplant

Mr. Lin was a 53-year-old chronic kidney failure patient who suffered from severe complications because of long-term renal dialysis. His son, who has blood type AB, wanted to donate a kidney to his father, who has blood type B. Following complete assessment and planning by the National Cheng Kung University Hospital transplant team, Mr. Lin agreed to an ABO-incompatible living-donor kidney transplant. To deal with the blood type incompatibility, Mr. Lin underwent laparoscopic splenectomy and plasmapheresis (separation of plasma from his blood for later transfusion) and took oral immune suppressants.

After the transplant, Mr. Lin's renal function normalized, and by 14 days after the surgery, he showed no signs of organ rejection. This was the first successful ABO-incompatible living-donor kidney transplant in southern Taiwan.

National Taiwan University Hospital

No. 7 Chung-Shan South Road
Taipei 100, TAIWAN
Tel: 886 2 2312.3456 ext. 5992 and ext. 1078
Fax: 886 2 2391.0708
Email: ntuhimsc@ntuh.gov.tw
Web: http://ntuh.mc.ntu.edu.tw

Established in 1895, National Taiwan University Hospital (NTUH) is an affiliated teaching hospital of the National Taiwan University College of Medicine. NTUH provides a comprehensive range of specialty and subspecialty services. The main hospital and two branch hospitals house more than 2,500 beds. More than 1,000 physicians, surgeons, attending doctors, and medical residents serve patients at NTUH. Most of the physicians and many of the staff speak English.

NTUH is Taiwan's leading hospital for cardiovascular surgery. More than 300 heart transplants have been performed at NTUH, with a success rate exceeding 90 percent. The hospital's mortality and complication rates for thoracoabdominal aortic stent grafting are less than 3 percent.

The **Fertility and Reproductive Medicine Center** at NTUH offers a comprehensive infertility treatment program. The center has treated more than 7,000 cases over the last 20 years and has achieved a high rate of pregnancy.

For cancer patients, NTUH offers a full range of services, including surgery, radiation, biochemotherapy, and molecular-targeted therapy of such conditions as non-small cell lung cancer, nasopharyngeal cancer (NPC), and advanced gastric cancer. Orthopedic medicine is also a specialty at NTUH, where surgeons perform more than 1,000 replacements of knee, hip, and ankle joints annually.

In 2003 NTUH received worldwide recognition for its management of severe acute respiratory syndrome (SARS) epidemics in Taiwan. That same year, the hospital reported the world's first successful use of autologous stem cell transplantation to treat NPC. NTUH also boasts the world's largest clinical trials of human papillovirus (HPV-008) vaccine for cervical cancer. The hospital is also a pioneer in testing interferon therapy for the treatment of chronic hepatitis.

More than 13,000 international patients received treatment at NTUH in 2006, approximately 2,400 of them from the US and Canada.

Specialties

✦ Cardiovascular disease

✦ Liver disease: hepatitis, hepatoma

✦ Infertility

✦ Arthroplasty for joint disease

✦ Oncology

Services Provided for International Patients

✦ Billing inquiries

✦ Counseling

✦ Doctor referrals

✦ Providing medical reports

✦ Scheduling of appointments

✦ Assistance with arranging airport pickup and transportation, flight reservations and confirmations, accommodations, and translation services

Achievements

✦ 1996: Asia's first successful artificial heart transplant

✦ 1998: World's first successful cardiac cryosurgery

✦ 1999: Asia's first microstereotactic deep-brain stimulation surgery for Parkinson's disease

✦ 2000: World's first successful use of skin stem cells for corneal transplant

✦ 2005: Asia's first successful positive cross-matched, living-donor kidney transplant

✦ 2006: World's first successful endoscopic potassium-titanyl-phosphate (KTP) laser surgery for recurrent nasopharyngeal carcinoma

Feature Story

Children for Liza

Liza is a successful career woman from Manila, the Philippines. She and her husband had been trying to have children of their own for more than five years. They tried various infertility treatments in the Philippines, including one course of in vitro fertilization (IVF), but none proved successful.

From a close friend, Liza learned about the Fertility and Reproductive Medicine Center at National Taiwan University Hospital (NTUH). She was informed that NTUH has a very high success rate in IVF and charges lower fees than many other clinics in Asia. Through the NTUH Web site, Liza contacted one of the hospital's IVF doctors, who gave her preliminary information about IVF treatment at NTUH and explained the procedures of ovary stimulation, oocyte retrieval, intracytoplasmic sperm injection (ICSI), and implantation of sustainable embryos.

Since Liza did not speak, read, or write Mandarin Chinese and had never visited Taiwan before, she was referred to the hospital's International Medical Service Center. An English-speaking nurse practitioner at the center reached Liza via email and grew to know her well, eventually accompanying Liza through a series of consultations, examinations, and laboratory tests at NTUH. The center's staff helped Liza find a suitable hotel to stay at during her treatment and helped arrange for her husband to travel to Taiwan.

During the course of Liza's treatment, the center's staff showed her Taiwan's famous night markets, shopping centers, and other tourist attractions, and she was also accompanied to a Catholic church that had a parish priest from her home country. Liza said she was surprised at the extra efforts extended to her by the staff, and she emailed them often to express her gratitude.

After the implantation of fertilized eggs, Liza and her husband returned to the Philippines. Several weeks later, Liza happily informed the center's staff that she was pregnant with twins. The entire IVF treatment cost her about US$4,000. Liza said such outstanding and efficient service was well worth the money and that NTUH made her dream come true.

Shin Kong Wu Ho-Su Memorial Hospital

No. 95 Wen Chang Road
Shilin District, Taipei City, TAIWAN
Tel: 886 9 6895.9595; 886 9 6899.5995 (foreign language hotline)
Fax: 886 2838.9463
Email: a003837@ms.skh.org.tw; a008626@ms.skh.org.tw
Web: www.skh.org.tw

Open since 1992, Shin Kong Wu Ho-Su Memorial Hospital is the youngest hospital in Taiwan to be DOH-accredited as a Medical Center. It was also the first hospital in Asia to use positron emission tomography/computed tomography (PET/CT) scanning for tumor diagnosis and the first in Taiwan to establish a **PET Center.**

Currently, Shin Kong has 921 beds, with plans for expansion to 1,200 beds. The hospital is composed of 35 departments, including internal medicine, surgery, medical imaging, health management, obstetrics and gynecology, pediatrics, and more. Specialties include cardiovascular health, cancer treatment, total joint replacement, stroke prevention, infertility treatment, and cosmetic procedures.

Specialties

✦ Health checkups (14,000 annually)

✦ Imaging: PET/CT, 64-slice CT, magnetic resonance imaging (MRI)

✦ Cardiac catheterization (3,200 annually)

✦ TomoTherapy

✦ Sleep examination

✦ Cosmetic service

✦ Infertility treatment

✦ Joint replacement

Services Provided for International Patients

✦ Arrangements for appointments, consultations, and medical chart reviews

✦ Language interpretation in English, Japanese, and Spanish

✦ Cost estimates

✦ Arrangements for travel and accommodations

✦ Senior nursing specialists to assist the patient through registration, consultation, and admission

✦ Prescription medicine specially delivered to the patient

Achievements

✦ 1995: Taipei Hospital Service Quality Survey First Place Award (nonmedical category)

✦ 1996: Mayor's Award for Labor Safety and Health

✦ 1996: Council of Labor Affairs Golden Safety Award

✦ 2001: DOH Medical Service Quality Competition Bronze Medal (administrative category)

✦ 2001: Taipei City Health Bureau Excellent Home Care Award

✦ 2002: DOH National Biotechnology and Medical Care Quality Award

✦ 2003: Executive Yuan Outstanding Anti-SARS Merit Award

✦ 2004: DOH National Biotechnology and Medical Care Quality Award

✦ 2005: DOH Medical Service Quality Competition Bronze Medal (nursing category)

✦ 2006: DOH Medical Service Quality Competition Silver Medal (nursing category)

✦ 2006: DOH Medical Service Quality Competition Bronze Medal (administrative category)

✦ 2006: DOH Medical Service Quality Competition Bronze Medal (medical technology category)

✦ 2007: Bilingual Outstanding Genial Hospital Award by DOH and TCHE: Promoting Bilingual Environment for Hospital

Feature Story

Brain Hemorrhage Treated Successfully

Mr. Kawazima, a 23-year-old Taekwondo athlete from Japan, experienced numbness in his left arm ten minutes after a competition and later fell unconscious. When he arrived at Yang Ming Hospital in an ambulance, he was in a deep coma. After initial emergency treatment, he was transferred to Shin Kong Wu Ho-Su Memorial Hospital, still comatose but slightly more responsive.

A computed tomography (CT) scan revealed an acute left temporal lobe dural hemorrhage, which was causing severe swelling in Mr. Kawazima's brain. A Shin Kong neurosurgeon immediately performed an emergency craniotomy, removed blood clots to relieve the pressure on the brain, and placed a pressure monitor inside the cranium. The surgery went successfully, and Mr. Kawazima was transferred to the intensive care unit (ICU) for close monitoring and care.

In less than a month, Mr. Kawazima regained his ability to recognize faces. His recovery proceeded well and he was transferred to a regular care unit, where he continued to make progress through rehabilitation. After a month of therapy, he was alert and oriented and could walk with minimal assistance. He was later able to return home to Japan to continue his treatment and recovery.

Show Chwan Health Care System (Chang-Bing Show Chwan Health Care Center Park)

No. 6 Lugong Road, Lukang Zhen
Changhua County, TAIWAN
Tel: 886 9 2188.8611
Fax: 886 2 2351.7988; 886 2 4707.3226
Email: brady@24drs.com; tobrady@gmail.com
Web: www.cbshow.org.tw

Chang-Bing Show Chwan Health Care Center Park is a new concept in healthcare design: a "health park" that integrates treatment facilities, an art gallery, a movie theater, and a museum along with restaurants, retail stores, recreational facilities, and convenient transportation into what its planners call "a unique and holistic healthcare experience." Show Chwan staffers meld a patient-centered philosophy with the latest medical technology, including positron emission tomography/computed tomography (PET/CT) scanning, robotic arm (minimally invasive) surgery, Gamma Knife radiosurgery, and more. Three packages of health and wellness examinations are available.

The hospital opened in 2006, with 1,000 beds and nearly 400 physicians and surgeons. It's affiliated with Johns Hopkins University Welch Center, Tokyo Women's Hospital, Vancouver General in Canada, and Garfield Medical Center in Los Angeles. Treatment specialties include orthopedics, cardiovascular surgery, gastroenterology, neurology, neurosurgery, and various cosmetic procedures. Many of Show Chwan's physicians and surgeons trained in Japan, Europe, and the US.

In 2008 Show Chwan opened the **Research Institute Against Cancer of the Digestive Tract** (ASIA-IRCAD).

Through IRCAD-EITS, ASIA-IRCAD is partnered with the European Institute of Telesurgery, one of the world's best minimally invasive surgery training and research centers (headed by Dr. Jacques Marescaux of the University of Strasbourg, France). ASIA-IRCAD is working toward becoming a major center for minimally invasive surgery in Asia.

Specialties

✦ Orthopedic surgery

✦ Gastroenterology

✦ Neurosurgery

✦ Cosmetic medicine

✦ Arthroscopy and removal of urethral stones

✦ Excision of subcutaneous skin tumors less than 2 centimeters in diameter

✦ Total hip or knee replacement

✦ Coronary artery bypass graft (CABG)

Services Provided for International Patients

✦ Airport or high-speed railway pickup and transportation

✦ Arrangements for accommodations

✦ Assistance before, during, and after hospitalization

✦ Flight reservations and confirmations

✦ Language translation

✦ Medical referrals

✦ Visa extensions

Achievements

✦ 2008: TJCHA New Hospital Accreditation as an Excellent Teaching Hospital

Taipei Medical University Hospital

No. 252 Wu Hsing Street
Taipei 11031, TAIWAN
Tel: 886 2 2737.2181 ext. 3329
Fax: 886 2 2737.4257
Email: ipc@tmuh.org.tw
Web: www.tmuh.org.tw

When Taipei Medical University Hospital (TMUH) was established in 1976, it started with 220 beds. In 1989 TMUH received ISO 9002 certification. The following year, it was recognized by DOH as a Class I Teaching Hospital under the category of regional hospital. It has since modernized and more than doubled its capacity to 569 beds with another 200 planned. A new building opened in 2007.

In association with multiple outpatient departments, TMUH's **Department of Oncology** offers comprehensive medical care for cancer, which may include surgical tumor removal, radiotherapy, pain treatment, traditional medical treatment, and more.

TMUH's **Breast Center** provides reconstructive surgery, oncological care, and radiation therapy. Equipped with the most advanced breast ultrasound and a dedicated breast magnetic resonance imaging (MRI) scanner, the center provides early detection for breast cancer and a comprehensive service for breast diseases.

Specialists in TMUH's **Minimally Invasive Surgery Center** provide a wide range of standard and complex surgical options, from general surgery to advanced gynecological, urological, orthopedic, vascular, and neurosurgical procedures.

The **Renal Dialysis Center** provides state-of-the-art hemodialysis technology and a warm and friendly environment to patients. Regular dialysis treatments are offered six days a week. Peritoneal dialysis nurses are on call 24 hours a day, seven days a week. TMUH readily accepts visitors to Taipei who need dialysis treatment.

Specialties

✦ Cardiology and cardiovascular surgery

✦ Gastroenterology and colorectal surgery

✦ Urology and nephrology

✦ Neurology and neurosurgery

✦ Oncology

✦ General surgery

✦ Breast surgery

+ Laparoscopic bariatric surgery

+ Orthopedics

+ Obstetrics and gynecology

+ Infertility and in vitro fertilization (IVF)

+ Ophthalmology

+ Otolaryngology

+ Sleep medicine

+ Pediatrics

+ Rehabilitation medicine

+ Dentistry

+ Traditional medicine

Services Provided for International Patients

+ Assistance with doctor visits, registration, and hospital admissions

+ Help with obtaining copies of medical records

+ Arrangements for hotel accommodations

+ Arrangements for interpreters

+ Arrangements for transportation to and from the airport

Achievements

✦ Various years: Symbol of National Quality, Sleep Center, Endoscopy, Periodontics, Radiation Oncology, and Hospice and Palliative Care

✦ 1994: Hazard Analysis and Critical Control Point Accreditation

✦ 1994: CNLA Certification of Laboratory Medicine

✦ 1998: ISO 9002/Healthmark Certification

✦ 2002: National Nursing Management Conference Shi-Chuan Award and Excellence Ring

✦ 2005: Taipei City Health Bureau's Best Healthy Hospital Award

Feature Story

Mother Gives Birth after Surgery for Uterine Leiomyomatosis

Mrs. Kung is a 31-year-old woman from Taiwan. She began suffering from severe menstrual symptoms in her youth, and these symptoms continued to bother her greatly into her adulthood. When she was diagnosed with a uterine myoma (a tumor composed of muscle tissue) at a clinic visit, surgery was suggested to relieve her severe bleeding during menstruation and improve her quality of life.

Mrs. Kung subsequently visited several other hospitals, at which each doctor she saw advised her to have her uterus removed as soon as possible — but she wanted to have children. Disappointed but still hopeful, she visited Dr. Wei-Min Liu in the Department of Obstetrics and Gynecology at Taipei Medical University Hospital. Following uterine artery ligation, 30–40 myomas were removed, and her symptoms disappeared soon after the operation.

One year later, Mrs. Kung completed a successful pregnancy and gave birth by Cesarean section to a healthy baby girl weighing 3.2 kilograms (about 7 pounds). She and her husband had their second baby in 2008.

Taiwan Adventist Hospital

No. 424 Ba-de Road, Section 2
Taipei 105, TAIWAN
Tel: 886 2 2771.8151 ext. 2843
Fax: 886 2 2711.5802
Email: ykko325@tahsda.org.tw
Web: www.tahsda.org.tw (hospital); www.tahsda.org.tw/pcc
(international medical services)

Taiwan Adventist Hospital (TAH) was established in 1955; it is one of more than 500 healthcare institutions operated by the Seventh-Day Adventist Church's worldwide mission system. TAH was DOH-accredited as a Regional Teaching Hospital in January 2007.

TAH specializes in infertility treatment, orthopedics, cosmetic procedures, and health examinations. Its **Priority Care Center** opened in 1989, and its multilingual staff provides medical services to the expatriate community in Taiwan. The center offers a relaxing, comfortable waiting area and an escort to and from all outpatient clinics. A VIP section in the inpatient department was established in 2007 to provide a private and comfortable environment for the center's patients who need to stay in the hospital; multilingual nurses work in this section to ensure that international patients encounter no communication barriers.

TAH is a member of the Adventist Healthcare Association, which is affiliated with eight other Adventist healthcare facilities in Japan, Okinawa, South Korea, and Hong Kong. It is also affiliated with Adventist Health Managed Care of Northern California (US), which consists of Loma Linda University and Medical Center, White Memorial Medical Center, Glendale Adventist Medical Center, and Castle Medical Center. Representatives from these hospitals meet regularly to share resources and discuss the latest medical advances worldwide.

In recent years TAH has hired seven physicians with foreign medical licenses to serve the expatriate community better and to develop long-term contracts with foreign medical insurance providers. TAH received an Excellent English Environment Award in 2005 from DOH and the Taiwan College of Healthcare Executives (TCHE) in recognition of its efforts in international medicine. TAH serves about 11,000 international patients annually.

Specialties

✦ Orthopedics: total joint replacement, total knee orthoplasty, total hip orthoplasty

✦ Spinal surgery: degenerative spine disorders, spinal disc disorders, osteoporosis disorders of the spine, metastatic lesions, spinal cord tumor

✦ Assisted reproductive services: assisted hatching technology, intracytoplasmic sperm injection (ICSI), preimplantation genetic diagnosis

✦ Physical exams: student visa, newlywed, senior citizens, life insurance, foreign residents, immigration (Australia, US, New Zealand)

Services Provided for International Patients

✦ Arrangements for accommodations

✦ Airport pickup and transportation

✦ Assistance before, during, and after hospitalization

✦ Scheduling of appointments

✦ Outpatient and inpatient service

✦ Bilingual staff, language translation

✦ Personal assistance from an assigned staff member

✦ Consultation by a full-time doctor certified by the American Internal Medicine Board

Achievements

✦ 1998–2008: Approved to administer immigration physical examinations for the embassies of Australia, the US, and New Zealand

✦ 2003 and 2005: Bilingual Outstanding Genial Hospital Award by DOH and TCHE: Promoting Bilingual Environment for Hospital

✦ 2006: DOH and TCHE Certification as a Baby-Friendly Hospital

Feature Story

Successful Surgery for a Stroke

After Ms. Wen became a mother in her late twenties, she, like many young parents in Taiwan, continued to pursue her higher education after work. One night as she was working at her desk, her husband thought her back looked strange. He checked and found her sitting stiffly with her eyes looking up, and she was unresponsive, so he sent her immediately to Taiwan Adventist Hospital.

Examination showed that Ms. Wen had suffered a stroke. She was transferred to the surgical intensive care department, where the neurosurgery department director, Dr. Huang, examined her carefully and diagnosed an arterial venous malformation blowout. Her condition was critical and her life signs unstable.

Dr. Huang originally planned to wait until Ms. Wen's condition stabilized before attempting surgery, but by evening she had received cardiopulmonary resuscitation (CPR) three times and her life signs were fading. Her husband begged Dr. Huang to do anything possible to save his wife, and Dr. Huang decided to operate immediately. Shortly after sterilization for the surgery, Ms. Wen stopped breathing. After the staff restored her respiration, the surgery began. The procedure lasted several hours.

A few days later, Ms. Wen awoke, remembering nothing of these life-threatening events. She eventually began rehabilitation exercises, such as getting off the bed and walking. She is now engaging in normal life activities, and her husband, who cared for her during her recovery, has been able to return to work.

Taiwan Landseed Hospital

No. 77 Kwang-Tai Road
Pingjen City 32449, TAIWAN
Tel: 886 9 1779.8922
Fax: 886 3 491.4000
Email: 1011@landseed.com.tw
Web: www.landseedhospital.com

Taiwan Landseed Hospital is only 20 minutes from Taiwan Taoyuan International Airport and a high-speed railway station. Landseed has 23 medical departments, six medical technology units, and two integrated comprehensive medical centers. Landseed is affiliated with 25 hospitals in Taiwan and 14 hospitals in mainland China.

This 750-bed hospital was established in 1995. It was the first medical institution in Asia to receive ISO 9002 certification for its quality management system and ISO 14001 certification for its environmental management system. Accredited as a teaching hospital in 2007, today Landseed averages 2,500 outpatient clinic visits daily and has served a total of more than 3 million patients.

Landseed offers a wide range of physical examinations tailored to a patient's needs and using the latest and most advanced medical equipment, such as 128-slice 3-D computed tomography (CT), to provide an accurate, safe, and speedy physical checkup. Such an examination can, for example, identify pathological changes (such as coronary artery spots, calcification, and narrowing) that could lead to a sudden cardiac crisis in people who are unaware of these conditions. A bilingual nurse is available to accompany international patients throughout the examination process. Specialists provide rapid and complete diagnosis, devise an individualized health management plan, and arrange regular clinic followups. The hospital also offers painless panendoscope and colon fibroscope examinations. Landseed opened a weight-management center in 2006.

Specialties

✦ Cosmetic surgery (intense pulse light, hyaluronic acid dermal filler, radiofrequency facelift)

✦ Health examination

✦ Dentistry

✦ Urology

✦ Cardiology

Services Provided for International Patients

✦ Arrangements for meeting with the appropriate physician(s)

✦ Arrangements for specific medical needs to be met while traveling in Taiwan

✦ Smooth admission and discharge at a single check-in/check-out counter

✦ Medical reports

✦ Followup visits/tests/reports

✦ Interpreter services

✦ Lodging and boarding arrangements

✦ Special diets as per patient's needs

✦ Regular supervision of all lodging facilities

✦ Currency exchange

✦ Travel and ticketing arrangements for patient and relatives

✦ Airport pickup

✦ Arrangements for sightseeing and shopping

✦ Local transportation arrangements for patient's relatives

✦ Prepaid cell phone card

Achievements

✦ 2000: Healthmark Medical Quality Management System Certification

✦ 2004: National Biotechnology and Medical Care Quality Award

✦ 2006: ISO 15189 Certification (International Quality Control)

✦ 2006: CNLA Accreditation

✦ 2007: WHO Health-Promoting Hospital Certification

Feature Story

Traveler Treated for Heart Attack

Mr. Santari, a 57-year-old American of Indian heritage, experienced heart pain, chest stress, and a cold sweat while visiting Taiwan. At the airport, a doctor at a satellite medical center operated by Taiwan Landseed Hospital used portable electrocardiography (EKG) to examine Mr. Santari. He was diagnosed with acute myocardial infarction (heart attack) and immediately transferred to Taiwan Landseed Hospital in Pingjen City, where he was treated successfully.

Mr. Santari's son wrote a letter of thanks for the prompt and effective treatment his father received: "Taiwan Landseed Hospital has given us an unforgettable impression. We would like to thank all the doctors, nurses, and everyone who helped my father and our family to overcome this difficult situation. Taiwan Landseed Hospital showed us that cultural and language differences cannot diminish the goodness."

Tungs' Taichung MetroHarbor Hospital

No. 699 Chungchi Road, Section 1, Wuchi
Taichung County 43503, TAIWAN
Tel: 886 4 2658.1919 ext. 4208
Fax: 886 4 2658.3311
Email: ttmhh@ms.sltung.com.tw
Web: www.sltung.com.tw

Tungs' Taichung MetroHarbor Hospital (TTMHH) is a comprehensive hospital that has been in operation since 1971. It has 1,405 beds and more than 50 subspecialties. Its specialized services include open-heart surgery, cardiac catheterization, radiofrequency ablation (RFA) for liver tumors, endoscopic surgery, and artificial joint replacement. The hospital's annual cases of neurotripsy and treatment of spine, tumor, and cerebral hemorrhage exceed 1,200. In addition, TTMHH offers complete plastic surgery services, health examinations, endoscopic ultrasound, and assisted reproductive technology (ART) with an in vitro fertilization (IVF) success rate of 36 percent.

TTMHH's **Health Management Center** provides personalized care designed to meet individual health needs. Multilingual coordinators to assist international patients, and examinations, followups, and consultations are arranged by the healthcare team.

TTMHH is an accredited teaching hospital certified for liver and kidney transplantation. It is the designated hospital in Central Taiwan for treating helicopter-transported patients and is qualified to handle "severe class" emergencies. The hospital cooperates with airlines to provide domestic and outbound medical services, international medical support, and overseas emergency transport for patients in nearby countries.

Specialties

✦ Cutting-edge medical imaging health examination

✦ Orthopedics: artificial joint replacement, endoscopic laser spine surgery

✦ Cardiovascular: cardiac catheterization, open-heart surgery

✦ Neuro-speed surgery

✦ Gastroenterology services: endoscopic ultrasound and RFA of tumors

✦ ART

✦ Cosmetic surgery

✦ Dialysis for travelers

✦ Personalized cancer treatment plans

✦ Dental implants

Services Provided for International Patients

✦ Comprehensive medical and surgical services

✦ International emergency medical support services

✦ Individual escort

✦ Multilingual staff and translators

✦ Airport and hotel pickup/dropoff

✦ Advanced, personalized VIP Health Examination

✦ Fast, efficient service (interim results within eight hours and final report within three days)

✦ Transparent price structure for all services and processes

Achievements

✦ 2004: Accredited by the Taiwan Society of Perinatology as High-Risk Pregnancy Emergency-Transport Response Hospital

✦ 2006: Accredited by the DOH as a Teaching Hospital

✦ 2006: Accredited by Taiwan Accreditation Foundation (TAF) for Medical Laboratories — Particular Requirements for Quality and Competence (ISO 15189)

✦ 2006: Accredited by the TAF as Alien Residence Certificate Medical Exam Hospital (to conduct medical exams for foreigners)

✦ 2007: Certified by the DOH to handle "severe class" emergencies (among the six such qualified hospitals in Taiwan)

✦ 2008: Accredited by the DOH for Hazard Analysis and Critical Control Point (HACCP)

Feature Story

A Child's Successful Open-Heart Surgery

Allan, a Filipino boy, suffered from congenital heart disease, resulting in slow growth and development. In 2006 with financial support from the Charity Association, Allan was transferred from the Philippines to Tungs' Taichung MetroHarbor Hospital, where he immediately received open-heart surgery to correct pulmonary valve stenosis and prevent heart failure. Cardiovascular surgeon Dr. Jeng Wei, one of Taiwan's best heart transplant doctors, noted that Allan's complex heart disease would have attained better outcomes if treated earlier. The surgery was successful, and the boy's condition stabilized quickly.

Allan improved rapidly after the operation, and the hospital staff threw him a party to celebrate his new life. He was discharged and returned to the Philippines in good condition. Allan's parents expressed heartfelt gratitude for the support their son had received, and Allan also thanked all his friends in Taiwan for giving him a better and healthier life. Tungs' Taichung MetroHarbor Hospital hopes to serve as a resource for many such critically ill patients.

Wan Fang Hospital

No. 111 Hsing-Long Road, Section 3
Taipei 116, TAIWAN
Tel: 886 2 2930.7930 ext. 7766
Fax: 886 2 2933.5221
Email: ims@wanfang.gov.tw
Web: www.taiwanhealthcare.com

Wan Fang Hospital is an academic medical center with 758 beds, employing 320 physicians and surgeons. Doctors in training at the university do their clerkships and internships at Wan Fang Hospital. Located near a major mass rapid-transit station in Taipei, Wan Fang Hospital has been operating since 1997 as Taiwan's first publicly owned but privately managed hospital. In 1998 Wan Fang Hospital was awarded the ISO 9002 International Quality Certificate. It received JCI accreditation in 2006.

Wan Fang Hospital is best known for neurosurgery, cardiology, orthopedics, infertility treatments, and laser cosmetic surgery (nearly 5,000 cases annually). Its **Laser Cosmetic Center** offers a wide range of dermatological treatments, ranging from Botox injections to microinvasive surgery for osmidrosis (secretion of foul-smelling sweat). Wan Fang Hospital's most frequent cardiovascular surgeries include cardiac catheterization and stenting (about 800 cases per year); other frequently performed procedures are open reduction and fixation of fractures of the extremities (more than 700 cases annually). About 8,000 international patients seek treatment at Wan Fang Hospital each year, most of them from nearby Asian countries, including Japan, China, Korea, and Myanmar.

Wan Fang Hospital offers a **CyberKnife Center,** infertility clinic, and cancer treatment center. The hospital uses specialized equipment, such as 128-slice volumetric computed tomography (VCT) for heart and virtual colonoscopy and magnetic resonance imaging (MRI) for high-resolution vasculography.

Specialties

✦ CyberKnife radiosurgery

✦ Spinal surgery

✦ Premium physical examination

✦ Laser cosmetic therapy

✦ Dental implants

✦ Cardiovascular surgery

✦ Joint replacement surgery

✦ Lymphedema therapy

✦ Weight-reduction programs

✦ Sleep disorders

✦ Traditional Chinese medicine

✦ Mohs micrographic surgery

✦ Minimally invasive surgery

Services Provided for International Patients

✦ International medical services Web site

✦ Arrangements for accommodations

✦ Assistance with flight reservations and confirmations

✦ Airport pickup and local transportation

✦ Assistance before, during, and after hospitalization

✦ Arrangements for direct admission

✦ Language translation

✦ Medical referrals as needed

✦ Scheduling of appointments

✦ Liaison with evaluation agents, employers, and insurance companies

Achievements

✦ 1998–2004: DOH Healthcare Quality Improvement Circle Golden Award (twice) and Silver Award (five times)

✦ 2003: Société Générale de Surveillance (SGS) Standards Certification

✦ 2003: ISO 9001, ISO 14001, and QM 9004 Certifications

✦ 2004: DOH accreditation as a Medical Center

✦ 2005: World Health Organization (WHO) Health-Promoting Hospital Certification

✦ 2005: Occupational Health and Safety Assessment Standards Series 18000 Certification

✦ 2007: ISO 22000 Certification

✦ 2007: Hazard Analysis and Critical Control Point Accreditation

Feature Story

A Brain-Tumor Patient from Palau Receives CyberKnife Radiosurgery Treatment

Miss L. from Palau, the Philippines, had been bedridden for more than a year because of a brain tumor, but the only treatment she could obtain in Palau was internal drainage to control the increased pressure inside her skull. Under the sponsorship of the International Cooperation and Development Fund, a medical team from Wan Fang Hospital went to see Miss L. in Palau; her diagnosis of a brain tumor was confirmed, and it was determined that the tumor mass was putting pressure on the brain stem and cerebellum.

With the help of the Ministry of Foreign Affairs, DOH, and Far Eastern Air Transport, Miss L., her sister, and the nursing director of Palau National Hospital came to Wan Fang Hospital with complimentary airplane tickets. First, Miss L. received surgery to reduce the intracranial pressure. She then received a series of four CyberKnife radiosurgeries. Wan Fang Hospital also provided her with a special walker to use during her rehabilitation.

Although she had been to several places in different countries for the treatment of her disease, Miss L. said that Wan Fang Hospital medical team was the friendliest and most professional she had ever experienced. When she left Taiwan to return home to Palau, Miss L. said she was grateful for the excellent care she received at Wan Fang Hospital.

Yuan's General Hospital

No. 162 Cheng Gong First Road
Ling-Ya District, Kaohsiung, TAIWAN
Tel: 886 7 269.3228
Fax: 886 7 213.4672
Email: cs@yuanhospinternational.com
Web: www.yuanhospinternational.com

Established in 1946, Yuan's General Hospital (YGH), located in the heart of Kaohsiung City, is a 645-bed facility recently TJCHA-accredited as an Excellent Teaching Hospital. YGH's mission includes both treatment and research, and the hospital is especially active in stem cell research, having established the largest stem cell laboratory in Taiwan.

YGH annually provides medical services to more than 648,000 visitors, with 55,000 entering via its emergency department and 20,000 as inpatients. Its specialties include treatment of digestive disorders and cardiovascular diseases. Other popular areas of expertise for international patients include reproductive medicine, joint replacement surgery, radiation therapy, cosmetic medicine, and dental implants.

Since the introduction of radiation therapy, the average three-year cancer survival rate at YGH has risen to 76 percent. Early detection exams using positron emission tomography (PET) and on-demand, onsite-manufactured radioactive contrast can accurately locate cancerous tumors as small as 0.5 cm (less than one-quarter inch) in diameter anywhere in the body. Other high-tech medical equipment in use at YGH includes a 64-slice computed tomography (CT) scanner, linear accelerator, TomoTherapy, and interventional magnetic resonance imaging (iMRI).

Specialties

✦ Cardiology and cardiovascular surgery

✦ Infertility treatment

✦ Joint replacement

✦ Digestive system diseases

✦ Radiation therapy

✦ Cosmetic medicine

✦ Dental implants

Services Provided for International Patients

✦ International medical answering service

✦ Communication channels available 24/7, including fax, email, and voice mail answered by professional associates

✦ Local transportation

✦ Pickup and dropoff services at the airport and high-speed rail station

✦ Coordination services for admission, treatment, and discharge

✦ Recovery facilities

✦ Bilingual environment

Achievements

✦ 1997–2009: Department of Health (DOH) Accreditation to Perform Assisted Reproductive Technologies

✦ 2005: Atomic Energy Council Medical Radiation Exposure Quality Guarantee

✦ 2006–2008: DOH Bureau of Health Promotion Mother-Infant Amity Certification

✦ 2006–2009: Taiwan Accreditation Foundation – Chinese National Laboratory Accreditation (TAF – CNLA) Quality System Accreditation on Medical Laboratories

✦ 2006–2009: International Organization for Standardization (ISO) Technical Committee ISO 15189 Certification (Medical Laboratories), to the Department of Clinical Laboratories and Department of Nuclear Medicine

✦ 2006–2009: Taiwan Laboratory and Inspection Body Certification of Compliance with Operational Guidelines for the Health Examination of Employed Aliens after Entry

✦ 2007: TJCHA New Hospital Accreditation as an Excellent Teaching Hospital

Feature Story

Teamwork, Trust, and Treatment

Muhammad Arifudin, a citizen of Jakarta, Indonesia, and first mate on an Indonesian commercial vessel, was rushed to Yuan's General Hospital's emergency department. While at sea, Muhammad had suffered an acute stroke that left the right side of his lower body paralyzed. He later developed sepsis — a life-threatening systemic infection — that caused his body temperature to spike and his breathing to become difficult.

Dr. William Lee was one of the physicians who first attended to Muhammad, whose condition was initially critical but soon stabilized. However, the patient's recovery depended heavily on his emotional state, and he was showing an uncooperative manner, largely due to the stress of being unwell and alone in a foreign country.

Mary Huang, the Ward 6A head nurse, quickly organized a treatment plan combining psychological and therapeutic practices. The chief care nurse, Nancy Wu, diligently coordinated the medical team as they earned Muhammad's trust and friendship, smoothing his road back to health. After a month, when Muhammad was well enough to be discharged, Dr. Lee said, "He is working his way to a speedy recovery. It is the teamwork of care that sees a good ending."

Katherine Kuo, a specialty nurse at Yuan's General Hospital, accompanied Muhammad on his plane flight home to Indonesia. This was not an easy trip for him, but she did her best to attend to his needs and anxieties. Because the feeding tube in his throat caused him to cough, Katherine had to assure other passengers that he carried no infection. She knew Muhammad would not use the on-board lavatory, so she advised him to wear an adult diaper. Throughout the six-hour flight, Katherine tried to relieve Muhammad's tension with big smiles, friendly small talk, and a countdown to the arrival time.

When the plane landed in Jakarta, Muhammad's wife and children were there to greet him. Muhammad and his family held Katherine's hands to thank her and the hospital for all the care and help Muhammad had received in Taiwan and on his journey home.

PART THREE

Traveling in Taiwan

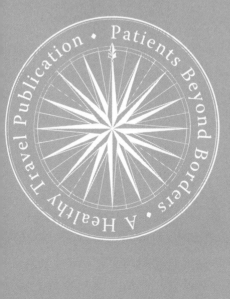

Map of Taiwan

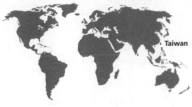

Taiwan

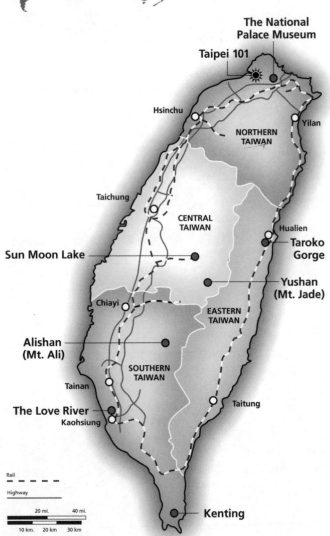

The National Palace Museum

Taipei 101

Hsinchu

NORTHERN TAIWAN

Yilan

Taichung

CENTRAL TAIWAN

Sun Moon Lake

Hualien

Taroko Gorge

Yushan (Mt. Jade)

Chiayi

EASTERN TAIWAN

Alishan (Mt. Ali)

SOUTHERN TAIWAN

Tainan

The Love River

Kaohsiung

Taitung

Rail

Highway

20 mi.   40 mi.

10 km.   20 km   30 km

Kenting

Healthy Tr

The Land and Its History

Taiwan is a beautiful island of high mountains, deep gorges, tranquil lakes, and offshore islets of every imaginable shape. Taiwan's total land area is only about 36,000 square kilometers (almost 14,000 square miles). It is shaped like a tobacco leaf, narrow at both ends. It lies off the southeastern coast of mainland Asia, across the Taiwan Strait — a solitary island on the western edge of the Pacific Ocean.

Taipei and Kaohsiung are the two major cities in Taiwan. Taipei is the capital and the nation's political, economic, financial, and cultural center. Featuring high-rise buildings and prospering businesses, it is an international metropolis bursting with vitality. Kaohsiung is the second largest city in Taiwan and a major industrial center. It is one of the Asia-Pacific region's most important commercial harbors and one of the world's four largest container ports.

Taiwan has a population of 23 million people and a population density of 625 people per square kilometer (about 1,600 per square mile). Among Taiwan's inhabitants, the Han people form the largest ethnic group, making up 98 percent of Taiwan's population. The other 2 percent include 13 indigenous tribes and other aboriginal minorities.

The history of Taiwan goes back 7,000 years. Pioneers of the Austronesian language family hailed from Oceania in different groups; they then became Taiwan's indigenous people. In the sixteenth century, the Portuguese discovered Taiwan. In the seventeenth century, the Dutch moved into Tainan and conducted colonial trade, followed by 200 years of a massive Han migration during the Ming and Ching dynasties of China. Taiwan then became a colony of Japan at the end of the nineteenth century.

After World War II, the governance of Taiwan was returned to Nationalist China. However, because of the Communist takeover of mainland China, Taiwan became a budding ground for democracy and capitalist economy, as well as a point of convergence for Eastern and Western cultures. This diversified history has fostered Taiwan's pluralistic culture. Indigenous peoples, early-era mainland Manchus, Dutch, Spanish, Japanese, Chinese, and American immigrants have learned to preserve traditional Han culture while simultaneously blending foreign influences.

Since the 1950s, Taiwan has dispatched agricultural mission teams to assist other countries' agricultural development. At the same time, Taiwan has received aid from foreign countries. As living standards improved over the years, Taiwan continued its involvement with international humanitarian aid. The development of the agriculture and livestock industry, the expansion of small- and medium-sized businesses, the sharing of digital and electronic media, and the training of medical personnel — all these achievements have demonstrated both the heart and the hard work of the Taiwanese people.

Historically named Ilha Formosa or "beautiful island" by Portuguese sailors, Taiwan is today a modern and developed democratic nation with a unique cultural heritage, enjoying the prosperity that comes from sustained advances and economic success in technology, industry, and science. In the past 50 years, Taiwan has undergone nothing less than an economic miracle. The nation now ranks in the top 14 trading countries of the world.

Southeast of the Asian continent, Taiwan is right in the center of the East-Asian island arc, bordering Japan and the Ryukyus to the north and the Philippines, Hong Kong, and Vietnam to the south. Thus, Taiwan is a hub that links the Pacific Ocean, South China Sea, and the Indian Ocean. Many airlines fly to Taiwan, making it an easily accessible travel destination.

Taiwan is suitable for traveling all year round. However, during certain traditional national holidays, in particular the Chinese New Year, which falls around February each year, many shops and restaurants are closed, and the island's roads are jammed as families return home for the holidays. In some cases, accommodation costs may double. We therefore suggest that you visit outside of these periods.

The seventh month on the Chinese calendar (approximately late August to early September) is the Ghost Month, during which activities such as traveling are taboo, so this is one of the quieter, less busy seasons in Taiwan. During this period the cost of traveling is relatively low, and temples often host interesting traditional festivals and perform acts of worship. You might therefore consider coming to Taiwan around the Ghost Month. Another good time to visit is in October and November, when the island's weather is pleasant and cool.

Because of Taiwan's geographic location between the latitudes 22°N and 25°N, its climate ranges from tropical to subtropical to subtemperate. Its ecological life zones are diverse and varied; they include oceanic, coastal, wetland, hilly, high-mountain, tropical, subtropical, subtemperate, and even frigid habitats for about 18,400 species of wildlife — more than a fifth of them rare or endangered — including the land-locked salmon, Taiwan mountain goat, Formosan rock monkey, Formosan black bear, blue magpie, Mikado pheasant, Hsuehshan grass lizard, and many more.

Continuous tectonic movements have created majestic peaks, rolling hills, plains, basins, coastlines, and other varied landforms in Taiwan. Visitors may walk along the cliffs of Taroko Gorge, ride on the Alishan Forest Railway (one of only three mountain railways in the world), or climb to the summit of Northeast Asia's highest peak, Yushan (Jade Mountain). Visitors can also soak up the sun in Kenting, Asia's version of Hawaii; stand at the edge of Sun Moon Lake; traipse through the East Rift Valley; or visit the offshore islands of Kinmen and Penghu. While preserving Taiwan's natural ecological environment and significant cultural sites, seven national parks and 13 national scenic areas offer numerous recreational and educational opportunities for nature-minded travelers.

The cultural aspects of Taiwan are also not to be missed. The blending of Hakka, Taiwanese, indigenous, and mainland Chinese cultures has produced a rich mixture of social and religious practices. Visitors can readily see the time-honored traditions of indigenous and mainland peoples intermingled with more recent influences from Spain, Holland, Japan, and modern America. Taipei's National Palace Museum has preserved the most comprehensive collection of artifacts of the Chinese cultures, organized chronologically and fascinating to see. Travelers may also learn about Chinese culture from visiting Taiwan's temples and other historical buildings. Traditional architecture displays a variety of folk arts, and temples serve as centers of folk culture and religious beliefs. For music lovers, theaters offer both local Taiwanese opera and traditional Chinese opera.

Taiwan's food aptly demonstrates the cultural mixing and matching of the nation's heritage. Situated at the convergence of world cultures, the island is an international foods paradise. Gourmets agree that Taiwan offers a fine selection of genuine Chinese cuisines, as well as Italian pastas, French dishes, German specialties, Japanese sashimi and sushi, and much more — even American fast food. The variety of fresh seafood from the waters surrounding Taiwan is something discerning diners do not want to miss.

With all of this richness, color, and flavor, it is no wonder that *National Geographic Traveler* praises Taiwan as "the best traveling destination in Asia."

Ten Things to Do in Taiwan

1. Eat xiao long bao (steamed dumplings) at Din Tai Fung in Taipei, ranked by the *New York Times* as one of the world's top ten restaurants.

2. Drink pearl milk tea (or bubble milk tea), a concoction of tea and chewy tapioca pearls. Many call this the greatest invention of Taiwan's tea culture.

3. Visit the Taitung indigenous tribes, the most distinctive native cultural group in Taiwan. Most of the tribes live in the mountains or along the east coast.

4. Visit Huatao Kiln, which works with four key elements — flowers, ceramics, kiln, and landscape — to provide visitors with a unique intellectual and aesthetic experience.

5. Visit Meinong, a Hakka town located in southern Kaohsiung County. Meinong is dotted with green tobacco farms and red brick-and-tile houses.

6. Visit Xiahai City's God Temple to seek your romantic fate from the "matchmaker," who is the diety of love with the appearance of an old man in Chinese tradition.

7. Take photographs in an art salon that offers creative and skilled photographic techniques. Create a memorable portfolio at a reasonable price.

8. Visit the Beitou Hot Springs region, comprising Hell Valley, Longfong, Fonghuang, Hushan Village, and Singyi Road. Jhongshan Road, Guangming Road, Sinmin Road, and Cyuanyuan Road surround the Beitou Hot Springs Waterside Park. The hotels in this area are large in both scale and number, and there's plenty to see and do.

9. Visit scenic Jioufen, which was once a gold-mining center called "little Shanghai" or "little Hong Kong." It is located in the hills of Northeastern Taiwan next to a mountain and facing the sea. Several movies have been shot there, and some have won international acknowledgment.

10. Study Chinese, becoming totally immersed in both the language and the culture.

Ten Unique Places
to Visit in Taiwan

1. Taipei 101—The city's greatest landmark. Located in the fashionable Xinyi district, Taipei 101 has become a symbol of the city's modernization and innovation. It combines Feng Shui with cutting-edge design. A high-speed ultramodern elevator whisks people to the upper reaches of the building within 39 seconds. The tower and its surrounding area are renowned commercial hotspots overflowing with high-end brands, such as Chanel, Gucci, and Coach, and offering a culinary paradise serving up all the cuisines of the world.

2. The National Palace Museum—For those interested in Taiwan's culture and history, the National Palace Museum is the ideal place to start. It houses the world's largest collection of priceless Chinese treasures spanning nearly 5,000 years of history. The Chinese Imperial Collection, beginning in the early Sung dynasty, constitutes most of the museum's 620,000 exhibited art objects.

3. Sun Moon Lake—Known for its high mountains and picturesque waters, Sun Moon Lake is the only natural lake in

Taiwan. The name comes from the moon-shaped southern part and the sun-shaped northern part of La Lu Island. Located in the middle of Taiwan, Sun Moon Lake is a great place for bird watching.

4. Love River — Transformed from a polluted river to a beautified area with parks and walkways lining the banks, Love River is a stunning Kaohsiung landmark. Love River's sightseeing boat allows visitors to take in the night lights while visiting the many cafés and art squares around the area.

5. Alishan — Originally built to transport logs and supplies, the Alishan Forest Railway has become an integral part of Alishan's recreational facilities. The railway climbs from 30 meters (100 feet) above sea level to 2,216 meters (almost 7,300 feet), passing through a cross-section of climates and terrain types.

6. Yushan — Yushan is the perfect place for nature lovers and mountain climbers. Covering 105,490 hectares (260,000 acres) of land, including large sections of the Central Mountain Range, Yushan National Park boasts a wide variety of plants and wildlife unique to Taiwan.

7. Kenting — Bright sunshine, blue waters, and clean sandy beaches make Kenting one of the most popular resorts in Taiwan. Kenting National Park offers visitors a profound and insightful ecological experience with its rich landscape of mountains, forests, pastures, coral reefs, and sand dunes.

8. Taroko Gorge — One of Taiwan's premier tourist destinations, Taroko Gorge is a gaping rift in the mountains, with sharp cliffs rising up from the riverbeds. The many hiking and mountain trails around this area allow full enjoyment of this magnificent environment.

9. *Danshui* — Danshui, named after a river called simply "fresh water," is a seaside town in Taipei County. The town is popular for its old streets and traditional snacks; it is also a great place for viewing the sun setting into the Taiwan Strait.

10. *Night markets* — For shopping and food connoisseurs, Taiwan's night markets are the ideal place to experience local culture. Enjoy 24-hour night life in "the island that never sleeps," taking in the all-night bookstores, discount outlets, and much more. Whether visitors are looking for street snacks or souvenirs, Taiwan's night markets are sure to dazzle and surprise.

Favorite Taiwanese Dishes

+ Oyster omelet

+ Coffin bread

+ Angelica duck

+ Rice tube pudding

+ Spring rolls

+ Stinky tofu

+ Deep-fried frogs with garlic

+ Bubble milk tea

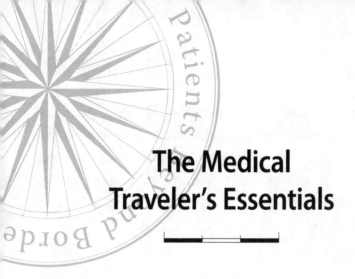

The Medical Traveler's Essentials

Language

The official language of Taiwan is Mandarin Chinese (Guoyu), but because many Taiwanese are of southern Fujianese descent, Min-nan (the Southern Min dialect, or Holo) is also widely spoken. The smaller groups of Hakka people and aborigines have preserved their own languages as well. Many elderly people can also speak some Japanese, as they were subjected to Japanese education before Taiwan was returned to Chinese rule in 1945 after a half-century of Japanese occupation. The most widely spoken foreign language in Taiwan is English, which is taught in the school curriculum. However, when taking a taxi in Taiwan, travelers should carry a note with their destination written in Chinese to show to the taxi driver.

Climate

Taiwan enjoys warm weather year round. The greatest fluctuations in weather occur in spring and winter, while summer and autumn weather is relatively stable. Taiwan is comfortable for most travelers, as the annual average temperature is 22° Celsius (72° Fahrenheit) with lowest temperatures ranging from 12° to 17°C (54° – 63°F).

Visas

Foreign nationals may obtain tourist visas if they hold foreign passports or travel documents valid for more than six months in the Republic of China for purposes of sightseeing, business, family visits, study or training, medical treatment, or other legitimate activities. Application requirements, the required documents, and other related items regarding visas are stipulated by the Ministry of Foreign Affairs. For more information, please visit www.boca.gov.tw.

Business Hours

Government	Weekdays	0830 – 1230
		1330 – 1730
	Weekends	Closed
Business	Weekdays	0830/0900 – 1730
Department stores	Open almost daily	1100 – 2130
Shops	Open almost every day except for the Chinese Lunar New Year	1000/1100 – 2100/2200
Convenience stores	Open daily	24 hours a day
Restaurants	Most open daily	Lunch 1100 – 1400 Dinner 1730 – 2100

Currency

The Republic of China's unit of currency is the New Taiwan dollar (NT$). Paper money comes in NT$2,000, NT$1,000, NT$500, NT$200, and NT$100 denominations. Coins come in NT$50, NT$20, NT$10, NT$5, and NT$1 denominations.

Telecommunications

Public telephones in Taiwan are divided primarily into two types, coin and card. Coin phones accept coins in denominations of NT$1, NT$5, and NT$10. For local calls, NT$1 buys one minute of phone time. Phone cards are available as magnetic strip stored-value cards, which sell for NT$100 each, and integrated circuit (IC) stored-value cards, in NT$200 and NT$300 versions. Phone cards are sold at railway stations, bus stations, scenic attractions, and convenience stores and can be used all over Taiwan.

When making local calls it is not necessary to dial the area code; for long-distance calls, however, the area code of the party being called must be entered first (see the explanation printed on the public phone) and then the number itself. International calls can be made from private cell phones, public international direct dial (IDD) phones, or hotel IDD phones (see also "Prepaid International Calling Card," below). Charges for international calls are applied in units of six seconds.

Prepaid International Calling Card

Prepaid international calling cards (or e-calling cards) are available for purchase at all post offices, the Taiwan Taoyuan International Airport Telecommunications Service Center, Mega International Commercial Bank, Hsiaokang International Airport, and various convenience stores. These cards are offered by different companies, and instructions for their use vary. Cards may work with mobile phones, but customers should check into their costs, which may include both roaming and card charges. For more information, contact the service center of Chunghwa Telecom at (in Taiwan) 0800 080.100 or visit www.cht.com.tw.

Country Code

The country code for Taiwan is 886. When making an international call to Taiwan from another country, enter the international access code followed by 886, then the area code, and then the number itself. For domestic calls inside Taiwan, the country code is not needed. Simply add a "0" in front of the area code. For example, to call TTFMT (in Taipei) from Kaohsiung, dial 0 2(area code) 2739.1322.

Useful Telephone Numbers

Emergency Numbers	Fire, Ambulance	119
(Free Service)	Police	110
Overseas Operator		100
Chinese Local Directory Assistance		104
Chinese Long-Distance Directory Assistance		105
English-Language Directory Assistance		106
Time		117
Weather		166
English Taxi Association		886 2 2799.7997
Tourist Information Hotline		886 2 2717.3737
24-Hour Toll-Free Travel Information Call Center		886 800 011.765
Taipei Foreign Affairs Police Station		886 2 2381.7475; 886 2 2381.8341; 886 2 2381.7494
Taichung Foreign Affairs Police Station		886 4 2222.3725
Kaohsiung Foreign Affairs Police Station		886 7 215.4342

Airport Tax

The airport tax is almost always already included in the cost of airfare for most travelers. If it hasn't been, visitors must pay US$10 as airport tax upon arrival. The receipt must be kept for validation when departing Taiwan.

Tipping

Tipping is not mandatory and is generally not expected, because most hotels and restaurants include a 10 percent service charge in their bill. If the bill does not include a service charge, visitors may want to leave a small gratuity for the service personnel.

Although tipping is optional, a small amount for bell service or valet parking is always appreciated.

Electricity

Taiwan uses electric current of 110 volts at 60 cycles. The type of plug is Type A, the same used in the US and Japan. Appliances from Europe, Australia, or Southeast Asia need an adaptor and a transformer. Many buildings have 220-volt sockets especially for the use of air conditioners. Many hotels also provide 220-volt outlets for British and European hairdryers, electric razors, and other appliances.

Transportation

Taiwan offers several convenient transportation options for both international and domestic travelers.

Air: Taiwan's international air routes are served by 34 airlines that fly to 56 major cities around the world. Four carriers operate domestic routes that reach all of the island's main cities and offshore islands.

Bus: Scheduled buses run from the airports to all major cities. Island-wide and regional bus companies also operate intercity services throughout the island. Tour bus operators offer buses for charter.

Taiwan High-Speed Railway (THSR): The THSR covers 345 kilometers (214 miles), connecting Taipei and Zuoying on the northern edge of Kaohsiung, passing through ten counties, Taiwan's four biggest cities, and 77 townships en route. There are eight stations along the line: Taipei, Banciao, Taoyuan, Hsinchu, Taichung, Chiayi, Tainan, and Zuoying (Kaohsiung). Another four stations, Nangan, Miaoli, Changhua, and Yunlin, will open in the future. For more information, please visit www.thsrc.com.tw.

Railway: Trains on the round-the-island rail network provide convenient services. Tickets may be purchased three days in advance. For more information, please visit www.railway.gov.tw.

Car rental: Cars can be rented at service counters in major airports, at THSR stations, and at a number of downtown locations. They may also be rented at international and tourist-class hotels, as well as from taxi companies.

Taxi: Many taxi services operate in and around Taipei. All taxis are yellow and display a light on the roof when vacant. The rate for taxis in Taipei is NT$70 for the first 1.5 kilometers (nearly a mile) and NT$5 for each additional 350 meters (0.2 miles). A 20 percent surcharge is added between the hours of 2300 and 0600, and a "waiting surcharge" is added for each three minutes when the taxi is stopped or is traveling at less than 5 kilometers per hour. Most taxi drivers cannot speak or read English, so providing a map or the destination written in Chinese characters is helpful.

Mass Rapid Transit (MRT), Taipei: The MRT system in Taipei currently has five lines in operation. The Taipei MRT, together with the metropolitan area's dedicated bus network, forms a convenient transportation system.

Since 2002 all local buses and MRT stations have accepted the EasyCard, a stored-value "smart card" usable for all modes of transit. An EasyCard is sold for NT$500, which includes NT$400 stored value and NT$100 refundable deposit. EasyCards can be bought and value added at MRT stations and convenience stores throughout Taipei City and Taipei County.

Please note:

✦ MRT running hours are 0600–2400.

✦ MRT fares range from NT$20 to NT$65 depending on the distance traveled.

✦ To provide passengers with a comfortable and safe ride, smoking, drinking, and gum chewing are strictly prohibited in MRT stations and trains.

✦ The use of cellular phones is prohibited in the first and last cars of a train.

✦ MRT tickets are valid on day of purchase only.

✦ MRT passengers are asked to carry pets in handheld cages; police dogs and guide dogs are excluded from this requirement.

For more information, please see the Web site of the Taipei Rapid Transit Corporation at www.trtc.com.tw.

MRT, Kaohsiung: The Kaohsiung MRT system uses the I Pass for travel throughout the seven counties and cities of southern Taiwan. The Kaohsiung MRT runs 0600–2300 daily. Fares range from NT$20 to NT$60 depending on the distance traveled. The Kaohsiung MRT system has the same rules and requests as the Taipei MRT system (see above). For more information, see the Web site of Kaohsiung Rapid Transit Corporation at www .krtco.com.tw.

Travel Agents

Credit: This content was provided courtesy of the Traveling Bureau.

Name	**Dragon Tours – Grand Travel, Inc.**
Details	Address: No. 167 Fusing North Road, 13F-2, Taipei 105, TAIWAN Tel: 886 2 2718.7300 Fax: 886 2 2718.0201 Email: service@dragontr.com.tw Web: www.dragontr.com.tw Targeted customers: American, European, Japanese, and Chinese
Services	Trip planning Transfer of medical records Travel and medical arrangements (airfare, hotel, hospital, surgeon/physician contact and scheduling, tour booking) Airport and medical appointment transfers 24-hour emergency contact number Pre-operative and post-operative counseling Assistance with passports and visas
Introduction	In business since 1958, Dragon Tours provides diverse services from basic travel arrangements to specialized medical travel packages for physical examinations or cosmetic surgery.

Name	**Lion Travel Service Co., Ltd.**
Details	Address: No. 170 Dun Hua North Road, 3rd Floor, Taipei 105, TAIWAN Tel: 886 2 2175.9888 Fax: 886 2 2712.1229 Email: lion@liontravel.com Web: www.liontravel.com Targeted customers: Taiwanese, Chinese in Hong Kong (China), Shanghai (China), Vancouver (Canada), Los Angeles (US), Sydney (Australia), and Auckland (New Zealand)
Services	Package tour Flight booking Hotel booking Event planning Passport and visa assistance Bus and land tour arrangements Taiwan High-Speed Railway ticket booking
Introduction	Established in 1977, Lion Travel Service coordinates flights, local tours, fine hotels, and medical treatments. With more than 20 branch offices in Taiwan, Lion can provide "one-stop shopping and nonstop service."

Name	**ZION TOURS**
Details	Address: 5F, 111, Chung Shan North Road Section 2, Taipei 104, TAIWAN Tel: 886 2 2586.6717 Fax: 886 2 2596.8569 Email: Stephen_wu@zion.com.tw Web: www.zion.com.tw Targeted customers: Chinese, Japanese, American and other Asian countries
Services	Services include trip planning, booking of flights, medical consultations, accommodations, assistance in shipping in medical records, and pre-operative and post-operative counseling. Arrangements of airport and medical appointment transfers, cell phones, 24-hour emergency contact number.
Introduction	Zion International is a full-service travel management company. The agency assists health travelers seeking cosmetic surgery, dental care, orthopedic surgery, and other healthcare services in Taiwan.

Name	**Everlight Travel Service Co., Ltd.**
Details	Address: No. 65 Nan-king East Road, 6th Floor, Section 3, Taipei 104, TAIWAN Tel: 886 2 2509.8555 Fax: 886 2 2506.9128 Email: taipei@yy.com.tw Web: www.yy.com.tw Targeted customers: All Taiwan inbound visitors
Services	Daily tours of Taiwan Tailor-made tours Medical and cosmetic surgery travel Corporate travel Domestic hotel reservations Domestic and international air tickets
Introduction	Everlight Travel Service, in business since 1975, has been rated as an outstanding travel agency by the Tourism Bureau of Taiwan. Everlight can arrange medical and cosmetic surgery travel plans for international customers receiving healthcare in Taiwan's leading medical institutes.

Accommodations

Name	**Grand Hyatt Taipei**
Details	Address: No. 2 Songshou Road, Taipei 110, TAIWAN Tel: 886 2 2720.1200 ext. 3502 Fax: 886 2 2720.1111 Email: ellen.chang@hyattintl.com Web: www.taipei.grand.hyatt.com Number of rooms: 873
Location	Situated in the heart of Taipei's business district, Grand Hyatt Taipei is near the World Trade Centre complex and adjacent to the Taipei 101 Financial Tower. The hotel is also a short walk from popular shopping malls and entertainment venues.
Nearby hospitals	Chang Gung Memorial Hospital (Taipei Branch); Cathay General Hospital (10–15 minutes' driving distance); Taipei Medical University Hospital (20–25 minutes' driving distance)

Name	**The Landis Taipei Hotel**
Details	Address: No. 41 Mincyuan East Road, Section 2, Taipei 104, TAIWAN Tel: 886 2 2597.1234 Fax: 886 2 2596.9223 Email: service@landistpe.com.tw Web: www.taipei.landishotelsresorts.com Number of rooms: 209
Location	The Landis Taipei Hotel is a member of the Leading Hotels of the World. It is located within the business and entertainment districts in Taipei, approximately 5 minutes' driving distance from the domestic airport and 40 minutes from Taiwan Taoyuan International Airport.
Nearby hospitals	Shin Kong Wu Ho-Su Memorial Hospital (5 – 10 minutes' driving distance); National Taiwan University Hospital; Chang Gung Memorial Hospital (Taipei Branch); Cathay General Hospital (10 – 15 minutes' driving distance)

Name	**The Howard Plaza Hotel Taipei**
Details	Address: No. 160 Renai Road, Section 3, Taipei 106, TAIWAN Tel: 886 2 2700.2323 Fax: 886 2 2700.0729 Email: howard@howard-hotels.com.tw Web: taipei.howard-hotels.com Number of rooms: 606
Location	The Howard Plaza Hotel Taipei is located in the heart of the city with convenient access to the comprehensive transportation network. Most of Taipei's tourist highlights are nearby.
Nearby hospitals	National Taiwan University Hospital; Chang Gung Memorial Hospital (Taipei Branch); Cathay General Hospital (10 – 15 minutes' driving distance); Wan Fang Hospital (25 – 30 minutes' driving distance)

Name	**Leader Hotel Taipei**
Details	Address: No. 83 Roosevelt Road, Section 4, Taipei 106, TAIWAN Tel: 886 2 8369.2858 Fax: 886 2 8369.2859 Email: ntu@leaderhotel.com Web: www.leaderhotel.com Number of rooms: 72
Location	Leader Hotel Taipei is located in the Gongguan Commercial Center adjacent to National Taiwan University. The MRT's Gongguan Station is close by.
Nearby hospitals	Chang Gung Memorial Hospital (Taipei Branch); Cathay General Hospital (10–15 minutes' driving distance); Taipei Medical University Hospital (20–25 minutes' driving distance)

Name	**Howard Lake Resort Shihmen Dam**
Details	Address: No. 176 Min Fu Street, Da Ping Village, Lung Tan, Tao Yuan County 325, TAIWAN Tel: 886 3 411.2323 Fax: 886 3 411.1212 Email: room-wt@howard-hotels.com.tw Web: http://shihmen.howard-hotels.com.tw Number of rooms: 83
Location	Located alongside the tranquil Shihmen Dam, Howard Lake Resort's design integrates Chinese classicism with modern Western aesthetics, using natural colors and materials to create a restful atmosphere.
Nearby hospitals	Taiwan Landseed Hospital (20 minutes' driving distance); Min-Sheng General Hospital (30 minutes' driving distance)

Name	**Taoyuan Hotel**
Details	Address: No. 269 Dahshing Road, Taoyuan 330, TAIWAN Tel: 886 3 325.4021 ext. 188 or 166 Fax: 886 3 355.4481; 886 3 325.1222 Email: hotel@ms3.hinet.net Web: www.taoyuanhotel.com.tw Number of rooms: 390

Location	Taoyuan Hotel is conveniently located near the Taiwan High-Speed Railway and adjacent to the Taiwan Taoyuan International Airport. A Carrefour supermarket and Mitsukoshi department store are nearby, only 5 minutes away.
Nearby hospitals	Min-Sheng General Hospital (10 minutes' driving distance); Taiwan Landseed Hospital (25 – 30 minutes' driving distance)

Name	**Hotel ONE, Taichung**
Details	Address: No. 532 Ying-Tsai Road, Taichung 403, TAIWAN Tel: 886 4 2303.1234 Fax: 886 4 3702.6666 Email: service@hotelone.com.tw Web: www.hotelone.com.tw Number of rooms: 202
Location	Located in the city center of Taichung, Hotel ONE is the tallest building in central Taiwan, offering its guests a grand view of the city's bustling streets. Travelers need about 2 hours to get to Taichung from Taiwan Taoyuan International Airport by car.
Nearby hospitals	China Medical University Hospital (5 minutes' driving distance); Tungs' Taichung MetroHarbor Hospital (20 – 25 minutes' driving distance)

Name	**Evergreen Laurel Hotel (Taichung)**
Details	Address: No. 6 Taichung Kang Road, Section 2, Taichung 407, TAIWAN Tel: 886 4 2324.2277 Fax: 886 4 2324.2233 Email: elhtcg@evergreen-hotels.com Web: www.evergreen-hotels.com Number of rooms: 354
Location	Evergreen Laurel Hotel (Taichung) is located at Taichung's main thoroughfare, just a few minutes from the National Natural Science Museum and the downtown commercial district.
Nearby hospital	China Medical University Hospital (20 minutes' driving distance)

Name	**Howard Prince Hotel Taichung**
Details	Address: No. 129 Anho Road, Taichung 407, TAIWAN Tel: 886 4 2463.2323 Fax: 886 4 2463.3333 Email: sales-tc@howard-hotels.com.tw Web: www.howard-hotels.com.tw Number of rooms: 155
Location	Located by the Chungkang Freeway Interchange, Howard Prince Hotel Taichung offers convenient access to all the science parks and industrial estates of central Taiwan, as well as numerous popular tourist attractions.
Nearby hospitals	Tungs' Taichung MetroHarbor Hospital (20–25-minutes' driving distance); China Medical University Hospital (30 minutes' driving distance)

Name	**Windsor Hotel Taichung**
Details	Address: No. 78-3 Taichung Kang Road, Section 3, Taichung 407, TAIWAN Tel: 886 4 2465.6555 Fax: 886 4 2465.8555 Email: windsorrsvn@windsortaiwan.com Web: www.windsortaiwan.com Number of rooms: 149
Location	One of a pair of twin towers, Windsor Hotel is a Taichung landmark, providing its guests with views of Taichung City and Dadu Mountain. Highways #1 and #3 are 10 minutes away; the Taichung High-Speed Rail Station is 15 minutes away. Taichung Science Park, Taichung Industrial Park, and Taichung Airport can be reached in less than 30 minutes.
Nearby hospital	Tungs' Taichung MetroHarbor Hospital (25 minutes' driving distance)

Name	**Tayih Landis Hotel Tainan**
Details	Address: No. 660 Shimen Road, Section 1, Tainan 700, TAIWAN Tel: 886 6 213.5555 Fax: 886 6 215.7766 Email: teresa@tayihlandis.com.tw Web: www.tayihlandis.com.tw Number of rooms: 315
Location	Situated in Taiwan's historic old capital, Tayih Landis Hotel Tainan is a short walking distance from sightseeing, shopping, and entertainment venues.
Nearby hospital	National Cheng Kung University Hospital (10–15 minutes' driving distance)

Name	**Evergreen Plaza Hotel Tainan**
Details	Address: No. 1 Lane 336, Chunghua East Road, Section 3, Tainan 701, TAIWAN Tel: 886 6 289.9988 Fax: 886 6 289.6699 Email: ceod@tscevergreen.com.tw Web: www.evergreen-hotels.com Number of rooms: 197
Location	Situated in the eastern district of Tainan, the modern Evergreen Plaza Hotel is located next to the Tainan City Cultural Center, Ren-De Highway Interchange, and Tainan Airport.
Nearby hospital	National Cheng Kung University Hospital (10–15 minutes' driving distance)

Name	**Howard Plaza Hotel Kaohsiung**
Details	Address: No. 311 Chihsien First Road, Kaohsiung 800, TAIWAN Tel: 886 7 236.2323 Fax: 886 7 235.8383 Email: rsvn-ks@howard-hotels.com.tw Web: www.howard-hotels.com.tw Number of rooms: 283

Location	Howard Plaza Hotel Kaohsiung is located in the heart of the business district with easy access to the railway station, a major highway, the Liuho night market, and other shopping areas.
Nearby hospitals	Yuan's General Hospital (15 minutes' driving distance); Kaohsiung Medical University Chung-Ho Memorial Hospital (5–10 minutes' driving distance)

Name	**The Splendor Kaohsiung**
Details	Address: No. 1 Tzu-chiang Third Road, Kaohsiung 802, TAIWAN Tel: 886 7 566.8000 Fax: 886 7 566.8080 Email: xsales.kh@thesplendor.com Web: www.thesplendor-khh.com Number of rooms: 592
Location	The Splendor Kaohsiung is conveniently situated near major land, sea, and air transportation centers, including Kaohsiung International Airport, Kaohsiung International Commercial Harbor, Shing-Kuang Pier, Ocean Star, Sun Yat Sen Freeway, and the R8 Kaohsiung MRT Station.
Nearby hospitals	Yuan's General Hospital (5 minutes' driving distance); Kaohsiung Medical University Chung-Ho Memorial Hospital (25 minutes' driving distance); E-Da Hospital (45 minutes' driving distance)

Name	**Kavalan Hotel**
Details	Address: No. 155 Gongzheng Road, Luodong Town, Yilan County 265, TAIWAN Tel: 886 3 956.8488 Fax: 886 3 956.8388 Email: kavalan_hotel@yahoo.com.tw Web: www.kavalan.com.tw Number of rooms: 80
Location	Kavalan Hotel is located in downtown Luodong, a short distance from the Luodong night market, train station, bus station, business areas, and scenic attractions.
Nearby hospital	Lotung Poh-Ai Hospital (10 minutes' driving distance)

Name	**Landis Inn Lotung**
Details	Address: No. 511 Gong-Jeng Road, Lotung, Yilan County 265, TAIWAN Tel: 886 3 961.3799 Fax: 886 3 961.3800 Email: landislo@ms45.hinet.net Web: www.landislo.com.tw Number of rooms: 68
Location	Located in Lotung, Ilan County, Landis Inn overlooks Lotung Recreational Park and is near Tungsun River Park.
Nearby hospital	Lotung Poh-Ai Hospital (15 minutes' driving distance)

Name	**Parkview Hotel**
Details	Address: No. 1-1 Lin Yuan Road, Hualien County 970, TAIWAN Tel: 886 3 822.2111 Fax: 886 3 822.6999 Email: judyhuang@parkview-hotel.com Web: www.Parkview-hotel.com Number of rooms: 343
Location	Parkview Hotel is located in the Meilun district of Hualien City, next to Hualien Junior High School and Hualien Golf Club. It is 10–15 minutes from the airport and railway station.
Nearby hospital	Buddhist Tzu Chi General Hospital (10–15 minutes' driving distance)

PART FOUR

Resources
and References

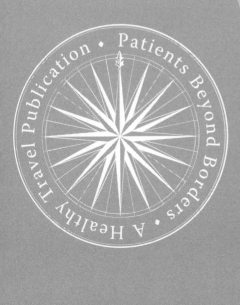

A Healthy Travel Publication • Patients Beyond Borders

ADDITIONAL RESOURCES

Other Editions of *Patients Beyond Borders*

Each year Healthy Travel Media publishes new, specialized editions of *Patients Beyond Borders*. Want to know more about Singapore? See the *Patients Beyond Borders: Singapore Edition*. Country-specific volumes are also underway for India, Korea, and Malaysia, as well as a treatment-specific series beginning with the *Patients Beyond Borders: Orthopedic Edition*. Visit www.patientsbeyond borders.com to check on special editions for your destination or treatment.

World, Country, and City Information

The World Factbook. Cataloged by country, *The World Factbook* — compiled by the US Central Intelligence Agency (CIA) — is an excellent source of general, up-to-date information about the geography, economy, and history of countries around the world. Go to www.cia.gov; in the left column, find "Library and Reference," then click on "The World Factbook."

Lonely Planet. This feisty travel book publisher has compiled a collection of useful online snippets (mostly as teasers to get you to buy the books) along with useful links. Go to www.lonelyplanet.com and search for your country of interest to find information on transportation, events, and more.

World Travel Guide. The publishers of the *Columbus World Travel Guide* sponsor the Web site www.worldtravelguide .net, which offers good information on countries and major metropolitan areas throughout the world. Go to the site's "Choose Guide" search to find information on airports, tours, attractions, cruises, and more.

Taiwan Sources

Medical Travel - Taiwan. The Web site of the Taiwan Task Force on Medical Travel (TTFMT), http://medicaltravel .org.tw, offers information on government organizations (including the Department of Health), the health travel industry, and medical institutions in Taiwan, as well as news and travel tips for international patients.

Information for Foreigners. The Web pages at http://iff.immigration.gov.tw provide information about visa renewal, residence permits, work, education, healthcare, taxes, and other matters for expatriates living in Taiwan. Visitors can search for specific information on the Web site, send an email to a government agency to request information, or call a hotline for personal service.

The Directorate General of Customs in Taiwan collects customs duties and monitors import and export cargo clearance and dual-channel (red-green lines) passenger clearance systems at international airports and seaports. Health travelers planning to carry items of value into or out of Taiwan should consult the policies and regulations at http://eweb.customs .gov.tw.

World Atlas

Google Earth. If you've not downloaded Google Earth, go there and do so. It's truly one of the wonders of the online world. After you download it, you can zoom to your home's rooftop or "fly" to any continent, country, or city on the planet simply by typing in the appropriate keywords. Legends include city names, roads, terrain, populated places, borders, 3-D buildings, and more. Go to http://earth.google.com/ and follow the download instructions.

Encarta Atlas. Encarta, Microsoft's easy-to-use, free atlas, allows you to quickly click your way around the planet and then obtain information on your country of interest. Go to www.encarta.com and click on the "World Atlas" tab.

Passports and Visas

Travisa. Dozens of online agencies offer visa services. We've found Travisa, at www.travisa.com, to be reliable and accessible by telephone as well. The agency offers good customer service and followup. Travisa's Web site also carries links to information on immunization requirements, travel warnings, current weather, and more.

Currency Converter

www.xe.com. To learn quickly how much your dollar is worth in your country of interest, go to the www.xe.com homepage and click on "Quick Currency Converter."

International Hospital Accreditation

Joint Commission International. Mentioned frequently throughout this book, the Joint Commission International (JCI) remains the only game in town for international hospital accreditation. To see a current list of accredited hospitals by country, go to www.jointcommission international.org.

Medical Dictionary

Merriam-Webster's Medical Dictionary. If a multisyllabic medical term stumps you, don't run out and purchase an unabridged brick of a medical dictionary. Several free, online medical glossaries offer more than you probably want to know on most health topics. *Merriam-Webster's Medical Dictionary* is provided on a number of sites, including MedlinePlus (http://medlineplus.gov) and InteliHealth (www.intelihealth.com). The simplest access is through http://dictionary.reference.com. Simply type in a medical word or phrase and voila! For a richer exploration of a given medical term, MedicineNet (www.medicinenet.com) and similar sources offer articles, services, and a thicket of sponsored links.

Medical Information

MedlinePlus is a US government-sponsored medical site that brings together a wealth of information from the National Library of Medicine (the world's largest medical library), the National Institutes of Health, *Merriam-Webster's Medical Dictionary,* the *United States Pharmacopeia,* and other sources. Go to www.medlineplus.gov and click any of the various choices in the left column.

The online tour at www.nlm.nih.gov/medlineplus/tour/medlineplustour.html helps you navigate this massive site.

Medical Travel Resources

Medical Tourism Insight is a monthly online newsletter written for the medical travel industry as well as employers, benefits managers, government officials, and prospective patients. Coverage includes objective and timely information on overseas medical care and related issues, such as health insurance and employee health benefits. The Web site is www.medicaltourisminsight.com.

The ***International Medical Travel Journal*** (*IMTJ*) is the world's leading journal for the medical travel industry. While it's geared more toward industry professionals than consumers, it does provide a free guide for potential patients at www.imtjonline.com. There's a free email newsletter, too, and a paid subscription service for those who are serious about industry news.

International Society of Travel Medicine. If you are looking for information about immunizations, infectious diseases, or other aspects of medical travel, check out the Web site of the International Society of Travel Medicine (ISTM), www.istm.org. This organization maintains offices in Georgia and in Munich, Germany, to promote safe and healthy travel and to facilitate education, service, and research activities in the field of travel medicine. Most useful to the health traveler is the society's searchable database of health travel practitioners.

International Medical Travel Association. Based in Singapore, the International Medical Travel Association (IMTA) and its small but growing membership advocate international patients' rights, quality assurance standards for international hospitals, excellence in continuity of care, and other patient-provider issues. For more information, email pa@westexcellence.com.

Beauty from Afar. If you're seeking more specialized information on cosmetic or aesthetic surgery or dental care, author and medical traveler Jeff Schult has gathered information on the main destinations, leading clinics and facilities, and third-party agents. Published in July 2006 (Stewart, Tabori & Chang), this 224-page paperback is written in an anecdotal style, providing numerous firsthand accounts that give prospective patients a thorough perspective on the health travel experience.

Medical Tourism in Developing Countries, by Milica Z. Bookman and Karla R. Bookman (Palgrave Macmillan, 2007), explores the international marketplace for medical services and its dollars-and-cents potential for developing countries. While it's more an academic work than a consumer guide, physicians, administrators, and healthcare officials will find this book's economic perspective and vast bank of data on the industry instructive.

1 888 STAR-012. Star Hospitals (www.starhospitals.net), a North American healthcare service, operates this toll-free call center staffed entirely by medical professionals. Staff members provide potential clients with guidance and information on member hospitals in India, Singapore, and Thailand.

A couple of magazine articles are worth a trip to your local library or an online search to dig up. If you are considering in vitro fertilization, you need to read "How Far Would You Go to Have a Baby?" by Brian Alexander, which appeared in the May 2005 issue of *Glamour*. On broader topics, Jennifer Wolff's "Passport to Cheaper Health Care?" assesses the pros and cons of medical travel. You'll find it in the October 2007 issue of *Good Housekeeping* or online at www.goodhouse keeping.com/health/cheaper-health-care-1007.

Web Resources

Medical Nomad. A group of medical professionals, technology geeks, and consultants established www.medical nomad.com in 2004 to bring together an impressive body of information, including specific data on treatments, clinics, physicians, accreditation, and other topics of interest to the health traveler. Medical Nomad's extensive database allows readers to search by procedure, provider, and destination, with clinic and country summaries as well as lay summaries of common treatments.

The Google Guide. While you may not wish to become a wild-eyed expert on the nuances of search engines, a little additional knowledge can greatly enhance your efficiency in narrowing your health travel choices. Consultant and Internet search guru Nancy Blachman (co-author of the book *How to do Everything with Google*) has posted a useful online tuto-

rial entitled "The Google Guide." Go to www.googleguide.com, click on "Novice," and you'll find a wealth of information on conducting Internet searches that will greatly improve your online health travel quests. Most of this information applies to other search engines as well, including Yahoo, MSN, and AOL.

RevaHealth.com is an Internet-based searchable database of healthcare providers. Its unique directory system and powerful search engine allow patients to find detailed information easily. The platform at www.RevaHealth.com also lets patients select providers and talk to them directly for a consultation.

Forums and Feedback

Health Traveler. Learn what other health travelers are saying and recommending, then share your experiences and suggestions at www.patientsbeyondborders .com. The authors and editors of *Patients Beyond Borders* invite you to join a community of patients who can help broaden one another's horizons and get up-to-the-minute news about a wide variety of health travel topics. You can sign in, go to the "Revisions and Additions" page, and post messages (anonymously if you prefer; your privacy is protected).

BIBLIOGRAPHY:
TAIWAN AS A HEALTH TRAVEL DESTINATION

An Overview of the Healthcare System in Taiwan, Hospital Care in Taiwan. Taiwan: Department of Health, January 2006.

Characteristics of Healthcare in Taiwan, Hospital Care in Taiwan. Taiwan: Department of Health, January 2006.

Chung, Oscar. "Tourism for the Health of It." *Taiwan Review — Healthcare*, February 2008:12–17.

Gao, Pat. "Healthcare for All." *Taiwan Review – Healthcare*, February 2008:18–23.

Comprehensive Medical Care Services, National Health Insurance in Taiwan Profile. Taiwan: Bureau of National Health Insurance, October 2007.

Jui-Fen, Rachel Lu and William C. Hsiao. "Does Universal Health Insurance Make Health Care Unaffordable? Lessons from Taiwan." *Health Affairs* 2003:22(3):77–88.

Surroundings of Taiwan, Hospital Care in Taiwan. Taiwan: Department of Health, January 2006.

Lives in the Balance: Taiwan and the WHO. Taipei: Government Information Office, April 2007.

MEDICAL GLOSSARY

Many medical terms are used in this book. The following is a list of the most commonly used terms. For further information, please consult your doctor.

Acute-care. Providing emergency services and general medical and surgical treatment for sudden severe disorders (as compared with long-term care for chronic illness).

Addiction. Occurs when a person has no control over the use of a substance, such as drugs or alcohol. Also includes addictions to food, gambling, and sex.

Aesthetics. A general term for medical treatments and surgical procedures undertaken to improve appearance. Such procedures include (but are not limited to) facelifts, tummy tucks, laser resurfacing of skin, Botox injection, cosmetic dentistry, and others.

Alzheimer's disease. A degenerative disorder of neurons in the brain that disrupts thought, perception, and behavior.

Anesthesia. Loss of physical sensation produced by sedation. Anesthesia may be given as (1) general, which affects the entire body and is accompanied by loss of consciousness; (2) regional, affecting an entire area of the body; and (3) local, which affects a limited part of the body (usually superficial).

Angiography. An x-ray procedure that uses dye injected into the coronary arteries to study circulation in the heart.

Angioplasty. A procedure that uses a tiny balloon on the end of a catheter to widen blocked or constricted arteries in the heart.

Arthroscopy or arthroscopic surgery. The use of a tubelike instrument utilizing fiber optics to examine, treat, or perform surgery on a joint.

Bariatric. Pertaining to the control and treatment of obesity and allied diseases.

Birmingham hip resurfacing (BHR). A metal-on-metal hip replacement system, surgically implanted to replace a hip joint. The BHR is called a resurfacing prosthesis because only the surface of the femoral head (ball) is removed to implant the femoral head-resurfacing component.

Bone densitometry. A method of measuring bone strength, used to diagnose osteoporosis.

Botox. A nonsurgical, physician-administered injection treatment to temporarily reduce moderate to severe wrinkles on the face.

Cardiac. Pertaining to the heart.

Cardiac catheterization. The insertion of a catheter into the arteries of the heart to diagnose heart disease. See also **angiography.**

Cardiothoracic. Of or relating to the heart and the chest.

Cardiovascular. Pertaining to the heart and blood vessels that comprise the circulatory system. See also **vascular surgery.**

Cataract. Cloudiness of the lens in the eye, which affects vision. Cataracts, which often occur in older people, can be corrected with surgery to replace the damaged lens with an artificial plastic lens known as an intraocular lens (IOL).

Colonoscopy. An examination of the interior of the colon, using a thin, lighted tube (called a colonoscope) inserted into the rectum.

Computed tomography (CT). Sometimes known as CAT scan. A noninvasive diagnostic tool that uses x-rays to provide cross-sectional images of the body. Used to detect cancer, determine heart function, and provide images of body organs. May be used in conjunction with **positron emission tomography (PET).**

Coronary artery bypass graft (CABG). Surgical procedure to create alternative paths for blood to flow around obstructions in the coronary arteries, most often using arteries or veins from other parts of the body.

Cosmetic surgery. Plastic surgery undertaken to improve appearance. See also **plastic surgery.**

Craniofacial. Relating to the head and face.

CyberKnife. A tool for radiosurgery that delivers precise high-dose radiation to a tumor. Can be used for tumors of the pancreas, liver, and lungs.

Diabetes. A chronic disease characterized by abnormally high levels of sugar in the blood.

Discectomy. Removal of all or part of an intervertebral disc (a soft structure that acts as a shock absorber between two bones in the back).

Electrocardiogram (EKG or ECG). A diagnostic test that measures the heart's electrical activity.

Endocrinology. The branch of medicine that studies hormonal systems and treats disorders that arise when hormones are out of balance.

Endoscope. A slender, tubular optical instrument used as a viewing system for examining an inner part of the body and, with an attached instrument, for performing surgery or detecting tumors.

Extracorporeal shock wave therapy (ESWT). A noninvasive treatment that involves delivery of shock waves to a painful area.

Gamma Knife. A form of radiation therapy that focuses low-dose gamma radiation on a precise target, such as a tumor of the brain or breast.

Gastroenterology. The branch of medicine that studies and treats disorders of the digestive system.

Genetics. The study of inheritance.

Gynecology. The branch of medicine that studies and treats females, especially as related to their reproductive system.

Hematology. The study of the nature, function, and diseases of the blood and of blood-forming organs.

Hemopoietic or hematopoietic. Pertaining to the formation of blood.

Hepatitis. Inflammation of the liver caused by a virus or toxin. There are different forms of viral hepatitis. Vaccines are available for hepatitis A and B. There is no vaccine for hepatitis C.

Hepatobiliary. Relating to the bile ducts.

Hepatology. The branch of medicine that studies and treats disorders of the liver.

Holter monitor. A wearable electronic device used to obtain a continuous recording of the heart's electrical activity. See **electrocardiogram (EKG or ECG).**

Immunization. Inoculation with a vaccine to render a person resistant to a disease.

Immunology. The branch of medicine that studies and treats disorders of the body's mechanisms for fighting disease, especially infectious diseases.

Implant. *In dentistry:* a small metal pin placed inside the jawbone to mimic the root of a tooth. Dental implants can be used to help anchor a false tooth, a crown, or a bridge. *In fertility treatment:* to place an embryo in the uterus.

Intensive Care Unit (ICU). The ward in a hospital where 24-hour specialized nursing and monitoring are provided for patients who are critically ill or have undergone major surgical procedures.

International Organization for Standardization (ISO). An organization based in Geneva, Switzerland, that approves and accredits the facilities and administrations of hospitals and clinics, but not their practices, procedures, or methods.

Intracytoplasmic sperm injection (ICSI). A type of fertility treatment in which a single sperm cell is inserted into an egg using special micromanipulation equipment.

Intrauterine insemination (IUI). Introduction of prepared sperm (either the male partner's or a donor's) into the uterus to improve chances of pregnancy.

In vitro fertilization (IVF). Known as the test-tube baby technique. Eggs are fertilized outside the body, and then embryos are introduced back into the woman's uterus.

Joint Commission International (JCI). The international affiliate accreditation agency of the Joint Commission, which inspects and accredits healthcare providers worldwide using US-based standards.

Laparoscope. A thin, lighted tube used to examine and treat tissues and organs inside the abdomen.

LAP-BAND System. An adjustable silicone band inserted laparoscopically around the upper part of the stomach, thereby reducing the food storage area of the stomach and promoting weight loss.

LASIK (laser-assisted *in situ* keratomileusis). A laser procedure to reduce dependency on eyeglasses or contact lenses by permanently changing the shape of the cornea, the clear covering of the front of the eye.

Liposuction. The surgical withdrawal of fat from under the skin, using a small incision and vacuum suctioning.

Lithotripsy. A procedure that breaks up kidney stones or gallstones using sound waves. Also called extracorporeal shock wave lithotripsy (ESWL).

Magnetic resonance imaging (MRI). A noninvasive diagnostic tool that produces clear images of the human body without the use of x-rays. MRI, which uses a large magnet, radio waves, and a computer, is used to diagnose spine and joint problems, heart disease, and cancer.

Mammography. X-ray imaging of the breast for detection of cancer.

Maxillofacial. Of or pertaining to the jaws and face.

Microsurgical epididymal sperm aspiration (MESA). Obtaining immature sperm cells from the epididymis (which joins the testicle to the vas deferens), in cases where obstruction in the genital tract leads to absence of sperm in the ejaculate. The recovered sperm can be used for intra-cytoplasmic sperm injection (ICSI).

Minimally invasive surgery. Any of a variety of approaches used to reduce the trauma of surgery and to speed recovery. These approaches include "keyhole" surgery, endoscopy, arthroscopy, laparoscopy, or the use of small incisions.

Myocardial infarction. Heart attack.

Neonatology. The branch of medicine specializing in the care and treatment of newborns.

Nephrology. The medical specialty that deals with the kidneys.

Neurology. The branch of medicine that studies and treats disorders of the nervous system, including the brain.

Neuro-oncology. The branch of medicine that studies and treats cancers of the nervous system.

Neuro-ophthalmology. The branch of medicine that studies and treats disorders of the nerves in the eye.

Neurosurgery. Surgery on the brain or other parts of the nervous system.

Obstetrics. The branch of medicine focusing on pregnancy and childbirth.

Oncology. The branch of medicine that studies and treats cancer.

Ophthalmology. The branch of medicine that studies and treats disorders of the eye.

Orthodontics. The branch of dentistry dealing with the prevention and correc-

tion of irregular tooth positioning, as by means of braces.

Orthopedics. The branch of medicine that studies and treats diseases and injuries of the bones and joints.

Osteoporosis. Thinning of the bones and reduction in bone mass, which increases the risk of fractures and decreases mobility, especially in the elderly.

Otolaryngology. The branch of medicine that studies and treats ear, nose, and throat disorders.

Pacemaker. An electronic device surgically implanted into a patient's chest to regulate the heartbeat.

Parkinson's disease. A movement disorder most common among the elderly.

Pathology. The branch of medicine that focuses on the laboratory-based study of disease in cells and tissues, as opposed to clinical examination of symptoms.

Pediatric. Of or pertaining to children.

Periodontics. The branch of dentistry dealing with the study and treatment of diseases of the bones, connective tissues, and gums surrounding and supporting the teeth.

Physiotherapy or physical therapy. The treatment or management of physical disability, malfunction, or pain by exercise, massage, hydrotherapy, and other techniques without the use of drugs, surgery, or radiation.

Plastic surgery. The branch of medicine focusing on corrective operations to the face, head, and body to restore function and (sometimes) to improve appearance (also called cosmetic surgery).

Polio (poliomyelitis). A paralyzing disease caused by a virus and characterized by inflammation of the motor neurons of the brain stem and spinal cord.

Positron emission tomography (PET). Also known as PET imaging or PET scan. A diagnostic tool that captures images of the human body by detecting positrons or tiny particles from radioactive material. Used to detect cancer and determine heart function; used most recently as an early clue to Alzheimer's. May be used in conjunction with **computed tomography (CT).**

Prosthodontics. The branch of dentistry that deals with replacing of missing teeth and other oral structures with artificial devices.

Psychiatry. The branch of medicine that studies and treats mental disorders.

Radiofrequency ablation. The use of electrodes to generate heat and destroy abnormal tissue.

Radiology. The branch of medicine dealing with capturing and interpreting images, such as x-rays, CT scans, and MRI scans.

Radiosurgery. The use of ionizing radiation, either from an external source (such as an x-ray machine) or an implant, to destroy cancerous or diseased tissue.

Radiotherapy. Treatment of disease with radiation, especially by selective irradiation with x-rays or other ionizing radiation or by ingestion or implantation of radioisotopes.

Reconstructive surgery. The branch of surgery dealing with the repair or replacement of malformed, injured, or lost

organs or tissues of the body, chiefly by the transplant of living tissues.

Rehabilitation. The process of restoring health and improving functioning.

Renal. Relating to the kidneys.

Rheumatology. The branch of medicine that studies and treats disorders characterized by pain and stiffness afflicting the extremities or back.

Stem cell. An unspecialized or undifferentiated cell that can become specialized to perform the functions of diverse tissues in the body.

Stent. A tube inserted into a blood vessel or duct to keep it open. Stents are sometimes inserted into narrowed coronary arteries to help keep them open after balloon angioplasty.

Tertiary care. Care of a highly specialized nature.

Testicular epididymal sperm aspiration (TESA). A surgical procedure to obtain sperm from within the testicular tissue.

Transplant. *Organ transplant:* the surgical insertion of an organ from a donor (living or deceased) into a patient to replace an organ that is diseased or malfunctioning; transplants are available for heart, liver, lungs, pancreas, kidney, cornea, and some other organs. *Stem cell transplant:* a procedure in which stem cells are collected from the blood of the patient (autologous) or a matched donor (allogeneic) and then reinserted into the patient to rebuild the immune system. *Bone marrow transplant:* a procedure that places healthy bone marrow from the patient (autograft) or a donor (allograft) into a patient whose bone marrow is damaged or malfunctioning.

Typhoid. An infectious, potentially fatal intestinal disease caused by bacteria and usually transmitted in food or water.

Ultrasound. The use of high-frequency sound waves in therapy or diagnostics, as in the deep-heat treatment of a joint or in the imaging of internal structures.

Urology. The branch of medicine that studies and treats urinary tract infections (UTIs) and other disorders of the urinary system.

Vascular surgery. The branch of medicine focusing on the diagnosis and surgical treatment of disorders of the blood vessels, excluding the heart, lungs, and brain.

Wellness. An area of preventive medicine that promotes health and well-being though various means, such as diet, exercise, yoga, tai chi, social support, and more.

X-rays. A form of electromagnetic radiation, similar to light but of shorter wavelength, which can penetrate solids; used for imaging solid structures inside the body.

INDEX

Specific treatments are in *italics*. Main
entries for hospitals are in **bold**.

ABOUT THE AUTHOR

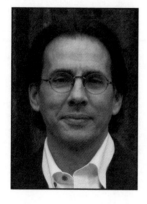

As President of Healthy Travel Media, Josef Woodman has spent more than three years touring 100 medical facilities in 14 countries, researching contemporary medical tourism. As co-founder of MyDailyHealth and Ventana Communications, Woodman's pioneering background in health, wellness, and Web technology has allowed him to compile a wealth of information about global health travel, telemedicine, and new developments in consumer and institutional medical care. Woodman has lectured at the UCLA School of Public Health and Harvard Medical School and has conducted seminars and workshops in a dozen countries. He serves on the Advisory Board of the Global Healthcare Summit and as Program Co-Chairman of the Global Healthcare Congress. Woodman has emerged as an outspoken advocate of global consumer healthcare and medical travel.